G000058508

What Your Doctor
May not Know . . .

What Big Pharma
Hopes You Don't
Find Out!

Disclaimer

None of what is provided here is intended to diagnose or treat any ailment. I am not a physician, nor should anything I write be taken as medical advice. I am simply reporting my own experience -- plus that which I have learned from books and several Internet sites. While I believe wholeheartedly in the curative powers of the ideas presented here, everything I have written is strictly a layman's opinion. Nothing here should be considered a substitute for the advice of your doctor. Rather, you should use it as a point of discussion with him or her.

I hope you find a heart doctor who is as open to this discussion as mine. While he has remained skeptical, he has been willing to monitor my condition and make recommendations. He was willing, for instance, to let me experiment with eliminating Lipitor (thank goodness) and stop taking two blood pressure medications -- both of which proved unnecessary. At this point, my doctor has read the two books I loaned him and at least skimmed other materials I have given him on this subject.

About those two photos on the cover and repeated throughout this book:

Both images are X-rays of my heart's arteries, taken during an exploratory angiogram conducted at Florida Hospital Orlando on July 27, 2011. I turned 70 years old in January 2012. Nurses in the "cath lab" said they hoped their own arteries right then looked as good as mine. The interventional cardiology specialist who performed the procedure proclaimed my heart healthy (*"free of obstructive disease,"* were his written words) as did my family doctor, based on the cardiologist's report.

The upper photo is of my Left Anterior Descending (LAD) artery bundle, commonly known to heart doctors as "the widow maker." At one point, it contained a blockage of 85 percent. Later, my heart became home to three metal mesh stents. The only damage this cardiologist could now find involved those stents.

The lower photo displays the clean arteries on the back side of my heart. That straight line is actually the X-ray image of the catheter that was inserted through my thigh, into my femoral artery and then threaded into my heart. Through it, contrasting dye was injected that would then light up the X-rays. Dark spots are intersections, where a branch attaches to the main vessel. They are dark because we are looking into the trunk of a wide open vessel, so the camera picks up a greater amount of dye in the blood passing through that point.

My change in heart health occurred *after* 17 years of bad reactions to every statin drug (Lipitor was the last and the worst). It was only after I had run out of statin options that I turned in desperation to searching the Internet. That's how I discovered the 1994 patent that changed my life. It might change yours, and that's what this book is about.

First Printing: April 2012

Special Note: Because this book was first created for e-readers in electronic book format, you will find Internet link references scattered throughout. I decided to leave them in the print version for those who would still like the option of looking up further information on the Internet.--DHL

INTRODUCTION

"Treating the symptoms of nutritional deficiency with drugs becomes nothing more than an experiment, where we get to observe the toxic effects on a malnourished body." – Author Unknown

My father's father died in 1941, a year before I was born. A doctor said he had "fat around the heart," and he needed to exercise. So he went for a jog, came home, and dropped dead at age 56 of a massive coronary. I have lived with that story all my life. In fact, every male in my father's family going back three generations has died from heart disease. My mother did, too.

I was just 48 when I got what I assumed to be my own death sentence. Tests revealed an 85 percent blockage in the LAD, my heart's Left Anterior Descending artery, the one doctors call "the widow maker." A doctor opened the artery in a procedure called angioplasty, by pressing the built-up plaque against the artery wall. But I spent the next twenty years of my life being cautious about exercise, and fearing "the big one." That fear is now gone!

By 2003 my heart disease had spread. In another angioplasty procedure, I was given three stents, metal mesh cylinders, to prop parts of my arteries open. And, on January 9, 2004, my then-cardiologist issued me a letter of "permanent limitation" of activities. He stated, "This patient has severe multivessel coronary disease and has undergone multivessel coronary angioplasty."

Yet, in a "final report" on results of my angiogram conducted July 27, 2011, an expert cardiologist reported my heart to be "free of obstructive disease." In fact, he concluded, the only remaining damaged areas in my heart involved those three stents placed there in 2003. A nurse standing next to him said she hoped her own arteries were as clean as mine. Reason for the procedure that day? Florida heat ... not a heart attack.

I had run out of hope around 2008, after Lipitor, the last statin drug available to me, ended up causing severe side effects, just like all the others I'd tried since 1989. I felt all I could do at that point was let my heart disease run its course until it killed me.

So, imagine my surprise when an extensive Internet search led me to U.S. Patent #5278189 – filed in 1994 by American scientist Linus Pauling and German medical doctor Matthias Rath. It claimed to be a cure for heart disease (technically titled "Prevention and treatment of occlusive cardiovascular disease with ascorbate and substances that inhibit the binding of lipoprotein (A)").

It's a patent Big Pharma, the American Medical Association, American Heart Association and U.S. Food and Drug Administration have all known about <u>since 1994</u>.

None of them has shown the least bit of interest. In fact, they have sought to diminish it and to denigrate its authors, one of them a two-time Nobel Prize winning scientist who had nothing to gain by its publication. There's no money in it. At least, there's no big money. This is an inexpensive cure based on over the counter supplements.

The two inventors placed their discovery in the public domain, and no public or private agency has even seen fit to give it an adequate clinical trial. Oh, they claim to have looked at it, but their questionable "studies" to date have been dismissive.

Yet, after three years on this regimen, my documented "severe multivessel coronary disease" is GONE – as in "<u>free of obstructive disease</u>," the interventional cardiologist's words in July 2011 -- and I am angry.

Why have I and millions of others suffered needlessly for most of two decades, when a cure was available? Why have so many of your relatives and mine died from an epidemic that could have been prevented? Why have so many suffered side effects of statin drugs? And, why will I have to live the rest of my life with damage caused by stents my heart never would have needed had this inexpensive cure for heart disease been widely supported?

As you read this book you will learn:
- Coronary Artery Disease can be reversed, cured and prevented
- cholesterol level is unrelated to heart disease
- statin drugs do not reduce death rates due to heart disease
- side effects of statin drugs are far more common than is being reported, and include permanent muscle damage, brain damage, loss of memory, and more.

Imagine the lives that can be extended, the suffering that can be prevented, when more people learn there already exists a safe and inexpensive cure for heart disease.

This book is for them, and YOU

January 9, 2004

Re: David H Leake

Date of Birth: 01/29/1942

OHC Chart #: 039138

To Whom It May Concern:

This patient has severe multivessel coronary disease and has undergone multivessel coronary angioplasty. When over stressed he developed angina because of disease that cannot be treated. At this time I feel he should work no more than 40 hours a week with a maximum of 8 hours a day. Pushing beyond this is too stressful for his medical condition. Please do not hesitate to contact me if I can be of further assistance. This is a permanent limitation beginning at the time of his angioplasty in August 2003.

Sincerely,

George E. Andreae, M.D., F.A.C.C.

GEA/mh

Copied from the original letter written by my then-cardiologist and re-sized due to format restrictions.--DHL

Table of Contents

DEDICATION

This book is dedicated to my Dad, his Dad, and all the millions of victims of coronary artery disease. Until my generation, none had a chance to beat this killer. Now, we do.

Special thanks to those who contributed their time and effort to helping me compile and edit this, my first book, and to all the experts who graciously permitted me to quote them.

CHAPTER ONE –

The End

Everyone likes to skip to the end of a book to see how it turns out. In this book, the end is so important I am placing it at the beginning.

When people learn I reversed my own heart disease they want me to cut to the chase. "How'd you do it?" they want to know, hoping they or a loved one can do the same. So, while I implore you to read the remainder -- to learn just how this works, and a lot more -- here is the secret formula.

1. Massive doses of Vitamin C (*as Ascorbic Acid*), 6,000mg to 18,000mg daily in divided doses. *Take with or before meals, i.e., 2 to 3 times daily.* At least for the first few weeks, take as much as you can, and never mind the FDA "daily values"; their silly 60 milligrams is enough to suppress the external symptoms of scurvy, nothing more. Linus Pauling, who patented this cure, along with German medical doctor Matthias Rath, was reportedly taking 18,000 milligrams per day to prove the safety of Vitamin C. He died at the ripe old age of 93, just a few months after obtaining his patent. Pauling's prescription for you, in phase 1: "Vitamin C to bowel tolerance," taken at 3 to 4 hour intervals.

"Bowel tolerance" level was one I did not want to tolerate, personally. However, I was able to take 10,000 milligrams, which I did for the first couple months. My maintenance level is 6,000 milligrams (the minimum recommended by Pauling and Rath) divided in three doses, morning, noon and night.

Vitamin C is absolutely the foundation for this cure. Taking anything less than 6,000 milligrams per day is cheating yourself – and your heart. You can buy it on line or at most local grocery stores or pharmacies. If you have difficulty swallowing the big 1,000 milligram tablets, try doubling up on the smaller 500 milligrams. That works for me.

NOTE: If "bowel tolerance" becomes an issue with vitamin C at levels lower than those desired, other options are available that might help. Non-acidic Ester C tablets are available in stores and on line. Liposomal vitamin C is said to be absorbed better; it, too, is available on line, or there are even instructions you can find on the Internet for the tedious – but less costly – process of making Liposomal vitamin C in your own kitchen.

2. L-Lysine 3,000mg to 6,000mg daily in divided doses. I take it with my Vitamin C. L-Lysine is an essential amino acid.

3. L-Proline 3,000mg to 6,000mg daily in divided doses. This was later recommended by Pauling, Rath and others to work in conjunction with Vitamin C and L-Lysine . If you are unable to find L-Proline locally, it has been available on line and at health stores such as GNC.

So, there you have the bare basics.

THE END (Just kidding)

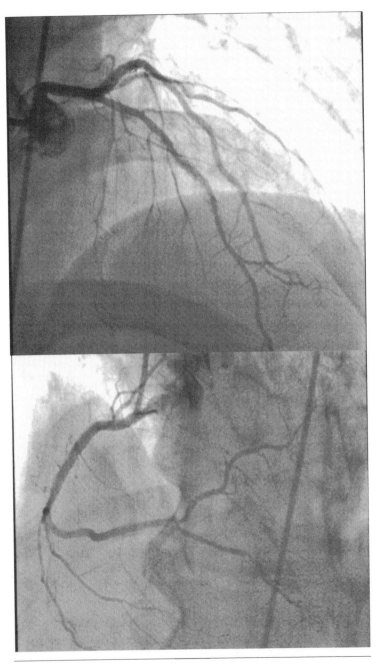

CHAPTER TWO --

Was Linus Pauling Nuts?

To my everlasting shame, I was not impressed with Linus Pauling when I met him. He was an old coot (63 at the time, seven years younger than I am now) and had only thirty productive years left ahead of him. Interesting, isn't it, how our perspectives change? He had an odd Oregon accent (i.e., distinctly NOT New England), and he wore that little poufy French beret. I was only 22 had just graduated from Boston University, and didn't know what I didn't know.

Our paths crossed in 1964, on the campus of Bowdoin College in Brunswick, Maine. I had been lucky enough to land my first job, as assistant director of news services, at Bowdoin. It was, and still is, one of the most prestigious small liberal arts colleges in the country.

That summer, the college opened its new dormitory for seniors, a mini-high rise tower dubbed, simply, "The Senior Center" back then. It was more than a dorm, though. It also housed suites for visiting lecturers – distinguished guests who would stay several weeks, and open their doors in the evenings for impromptu gatherings of students, faculty and staff.

Linus Pauling was one of the very first guest lecturers when classes began that fall. I was introduced to him at a party honoring his arrival, and we would pass occasionally on the campus pathways. He always sported that beret, and was usually walking with an entourage of Bowdoin's brightest science majors.

I heard him speak once. Gibberish, it seemed to me, because he was speaking in the language of brilliant scholars. My all-time favorite cartoon from the *New Yorker* magazine sums it up best; it depicted a scholarly gent looking at a blue collar Joe, and the caption read, "I'd love to explain it to you in Layman's Language, *but I don't know any Layman's Language.*"

That was the gulf between me and Linus Pauling. It was my shortcoming, not his.

At the time of his death in 1994, Pauling held as many as 48 honorary Ph.D.s. Wikipedia reports, "Pauling is one of only four individuals to have won more than one Nobel Prize. He is one of only two people awarded Nobel Prizes in different fields (the Chemistry and Peace prizes), the other being Marie Curie (the Chemistry and Physics prizes), and(he is) the only person (ever) awarded two un-shared (Nobel) prizes."

Quoting, again, from Wikipedia, "Pauling was in-cluded in a list of the 20 greatest scientists of all time by the magazine New Scientist, with Albert Einstein being the only other scientist from the twentieth century on the list. Gautam R. Desiraju, the author of the Millennium Essay in Nature, claimed that Pauling was one of the greatest thinkers and vision-aries of the millennium, along with Galileo, New-ton, and Einstein. Pauling is notable for the di-versity of his interests: quantum mechanics, inor-ganic chemistry, organic chemistry, protein struc-ture, molecular biology, and medicine. In all these fields, and especially on the boundaries between them, he made decisive contributions. His work on chemical bonding marks the beginning of modern quantum chemistry, and many of his contributions like hybridization and electronegativity have be-come part of standard chemistry textbooks."

No wonder I couldn't understand him.

However, in the mid-1970's, when I was suffering from back-to-back colds, I turned to a new book for help. It was Pauling's *Vitamin C and the Common Cold*, later re-issued as *Vitamin C, the Common Cold and the Flu*. I remembered the man I had met a dozen years earlier. By then I was more aware of his fame and his intellect. I expected his book would help me, and did it ever!

I began taking low doses of Vitamin C as Pauling recommended, and my colds went away. I have seldom had as much as a sniffle since. Little wonder, then, that my mind was open to his ideas when I came across his name again in 2007.

It was in the 1970's, also, that Pauling began investigating with several medical doctors the effects of vitamin C in extending the lives of terminal cancer patients – those hopeless souls whose diseases had been declared "untreatable." Their findings indicated terminal patients on chemotherapy alone died in about six months, while those terminal cancer patients who took only very high doses of Vitamin C remained alive 1 to 12 years longer.

Their studies were replicated in Scotland, Canada and Japan. Cancer treatment medications have improved since then, so their effectiveness might be better than vitamin C in most cases today. Still, there are cancer *patients hoping to gain time by taking massive doses of vitamin C.

All this talk about the benefits of Vitamin C was of great concern to the pharmaceutical industry (more on this in Chapters Three, Six and Seven). Perhaps it was because profits to be made producing natural Vitamin C are woefully less than those to be had from patentable synthetic drugs. It was at that point they began a campaign to discredit Pauling and other advocates for vitamin C.

It seems odd Pauling's competence could be challenged beginning in the 1970's, yet as late as 1990 he was still giving recorded interviews (some available on YouTube) about his ongoing studies of the atomic nucleus.

View one of the last known videos of him at age 93, shortly before his death, and decide for yourself: **http://www.youtube.com/watch?v=A5dba4DK0e4**.

More information on efforts to discredit Pauling can be seen at **http://www.cancertutor.com/WarBetween/War_Pauling.html**

Pauling was born February 28, 1901, in Portland, Oregon. He died of prostate cancer on August 19, 1994, in Big Sur, CA. He is buried in Oswego Pioneer Cemetery, Lake Oswego, OR, near where he lived as a child.

To answer my own question, No, I do not think Linus Pauling was nuts.

*(Note: Vitamin C's potential for treating some forms of cancer is on the front burner again – at least in non-pharmaceutical circles. A team of British researchers documented that taking massive oral doses of vitamin C can, indeed, increase its concentrations in your blood stream, far beyond levels previously thought to be the maximum possible. Writing in the Journal of Nutritional and Environmental Medicine in 2008 they reported: ". . . a short *in vitro* treatment of human Burkitt's lymphoma cells with ascorbate, at 400 μm L, has been shown to result in ~ 50% cancer cell death. Using frequent oral doses, an equivalent plasma level could be sustained indefinitely. Thus, oral vitamin C has potential for use as a non-toxic, sustainable, therapeutic agent."

Read more at **http://informahealthcare.com/doi/abs /10.1080/13590840802305423**.)

CHAPTER THREE --

What did Pauling and Rath learn about Heart Disease?

What if everything you thought you knew about heart disease was *wrong*?

What if cholesterol was not "good" or "bad?"

What if LDL was a life saving friend, not "the enemy?"

What if something else accounted for atherosclerotic blockages, i.e. "heart disease?"

What if you didn't need any toxic drugs to stop, reverse, or prevent heart disease, and maybe even prevent strokes?

In the early 1900's, medicine was at a crossroads. Natural healers, "naturopaths," believed in warding off disease by strengthening the body through the use of herbs and minerals, among other things. A lot of what they practiced – blood letting, poultices, and reliance on various natural ingredients – could only be explained as tradition. It was a form of medicine passed down through generations.

Medical doctors (M.D.'s) and laboratory scientists, meanwhile, were moving toward the use of patentable synthetic chemicals to treat disease. With the advent of penicillin and other "miracle drugs" during WWII the big money went into pharmaceuticals. By the 1950's, the American Medical Association and "Big Pharma" were waging campaigns to wipe out naturopathic "heretics." By the late 50's, naturopathy was licensed in only five states.

That was the way things stood until the 1970's, when a third front in human health care opened. Call it a new approach or perhaps naturopathy on steroids. Pauling coined a term for it: "Orthomolecular Nutrition" (see **http://www.ortho-molecular.org/index.shtml**). At any rate, a champion came along, one supporting an alternative to reliance only on synthetic pharmaceuticals to cure some of our ills.

This was no lightweight 1900's snake oil pusher. It was, instead, double Nobel Prize winner (1954 and 1962) Linus Pauling. He was among the first to start work in the field of *quantum chemistry* (**http://en-.wikipedia.org/wiki/Quantum_chemistry** and also in *molecular biology* (**http://en.wikipedia.org/wiki/Molecular_biology**.

Pauling was a scientist with impeccable credentials. He took us into the inner workings of the trillions of individual cells that make up our bodies. He was able to explain -- in scientific terms, not old-time hocus pocus -- how keeping all of those individual cells healthy could strengthen every organ and keep our whole bodies healthy. And, he explored alternatives to treating some of our most serious diseases.

As Linus Pauling explains in his 1986 book, *How to Live Longer and Feel Better*, "The world of today is different from that of one hundred years ago. We now have a much greater understanding of nature than our grandparents had. We have entered the atomic age, the electronic age, the nuclear age, the age of jet planes, television, and modern medicine and its wonder drugs. For the good of our health, we should also recognize that this is the age of vitamins." Going further, Pauling asserts, "The discovery of vitamins during the first third of the twentieth century and the recognition that they are essential elements of a healthy diet was one of the most important contributions to health ever made. Of equal importance was the recognition, about twenty years ago, that the optimum intakes of several of the vitamins, far larger than the usually recommended intakes, lead to further improvement in health, greater protection against many diseases, and enhanced effectiveness in the therapy of diseases. **The potency of vitamin C and other vitamins is explained by the new understanding that they function principally by strengthening the natural protective mechanisms of the body, espe-cially the immune system.**"(emphasis mine — DHL)

Beginning back in the 1970's, the medical and pharmaceutical "establishment" took a dim view – and still does – of Linus Pauling's work. Here was this brilliant scientist explaining how the body functions -- one cell at a time. When he then turned his attention to heart disease, he was talking about the curative powers of *inexpensive vitamins*. He was a threat to their line of reasoning, and to their profits.

The war for our hearts, minds and wallets was on. It was the altruist against Big Phama, the American Medical Association, and sometimes the U.S. Food and Drug Administration. We, the patients, have not stood much of a chance.

On one side stands the mighty conventional "Lipid Theory" of heart disease. Big Phama and the medical establishment employ an arsenal of patented (and therefore expensive) synthetic chemicals including statin drugs – along with invasive procedures ranging from stents to bypass surgery – *to combat a symptom* -- "the enemy" -- cholesterol. You cannot escape their constant advertising claims in the media.

The "Unified Theory" of heart disease, created and patented by Pauling and German doctor Matthias Rath, MD (**http://www4.dr-rath-foundation.org/**), stands in opposition. It has neither advertising budget nor a legion of sales weasels. It sees cholesterol as a *vital friend* to our bodies. It looks to restore heart health (horror of horrors!) *without the use of prescription drugs*. Its forces consist of a small army of believers – people like me, who have been lucky enough to learn about it, practice it, and enjoy restored health because of it. Those photos of my arteries on the cover – and throughout this book -- are, quite literally, living proof.

---------- ---------- ----------

When you look at another human being – or even yourself in a mirror – you see another human being. Medical scientists like Pauling and Rath see a complex assemblage of about 100 trillion individual living cells.

The cell is the smallest unit of life that is classified as a living thing. Cells are the building blocks for every organ in your body. Cells live, die and get replaced over and over again throughout your lifetime. And cells can get sick. Pauling was intrigued by the possibility of keeping cells healthy as a way of improving human health.

Rath has carried on Pauling's interest in this field, but has become the focus of establishment derision because on occasion he has overreached. He attempted to cure AIDS (as Pauling himself had suggested) in South Africa, for instance, using vitamins in hopes of helping cells fight off the disease. His experiments did not seem to work, several people in the study group died, and Rath and his program were banned.

Meanwhile, back to heart disease.

Using data they got from literally hundreds of published research papers by world-class scientists (MDs and PhDs), Pauling and Rath observed a link between cardiovascular disease and vitamin C. They would build on this knowledge to form their "Unified Theory of Human Cardiovascular Disease." The Unified Theory describes how the human body exactly regulates blood concentrations of cholesterol; it offers a compelling argument that, with proper nutrition (and not drugs) cardiovascular disease can be prevented and even reversed.

Healthy cells, both Pauling and Rath reasoned, could better fight off disease and resist organ fatigue. Pauling was particularly interested in the role vitamin C plays in the health of cells. In his 1970 book, *Vitamin C and the Common Cold,* Pauling advanced the idea that major doses of vitamin C could benefit human health. He was beginning to formulate his concept that many human illnesses could be traced back to a hidden, low-level version of *scurvy*.

Quoting from the website, Wikipedia, "Scurvy is a disease resulting from a deficiency of vitamin C, which is required for the synthesis of collagen in humans. ... Scurvy often presents itself initially as symptoms of malaise and lethargy, followed by formation of spots on the skin, spongy gums, and bleeding from the mucous membranes. Spots are most abundant on the thighs and legs, and a person with the ailment looks pale, feels depressed, and is partially immobilized. As scurvy advances, there can be open, suppurating wounds, loss of teeth, jaundice, fever, neuropathy and death."

In *How to Live Longer and Feel Better*, Pauling recalls the history of scurvy, once considered a plague of mankind. Between July 9, 1497 and May 30, 1498, for instance, explorer Vasco da Gama lost 100 of his 160-man crew to the disease. In 1577 a Spanish galleon was discovered adrift, its entire crew killed by scurvy. In 1741, Pauling reports, a British squadron of six ships lost half its sailors, dead from scurvy. Many California Gold Rush miners died of scurvy, too.

The British, Pauling says, were first to realize that fresh fruits and vegetables could prevent or reduce this disease. Keeping fruits or vegetables from spoiling on long sea voyages, though, was a problem, until they hit on lemons and limes. Eventually, every British sailor was issued daily rations of lime juice. They became known as "Limeys," a label that would stick through the ages.

It would be years later before research would reveal the reason lime juice worked. It contained a high concentration of ascorbic acid (vitamin C).

Another incident Pauling recalls riveted his attention on *invisible* forms of low-level scurvy … and the curative powers of vitamin C to strengthen blood vessels throughout the body:

"E. Cheraskin, W.M. Ringsdorf, Jr., and E.L. Sisley in their book, *The Vitamin C Connection* (1983)," Pauling reports, "recount the story of a forty-eight-year-old woman in California who came to the hospital because of pain, indigestion, and swelling of the abdomen. Over a period of four years she had six surgical operations. Each time the abdomen was found to be full of blood. In the effort to prevent the recurrent bleeding, her ovaries, uterus, appendix, spleen and part of the small intestine were removed. Finally, after four years, a doctor asked her what she ate and found that her diet contained essentially no fruits or vegetables and that she took no supplementary vitamins. She was getting a little vitamin C in her food, enough to keep her from dying of scurvy but not a sufficient amount to keep her blood vessels strong enough to prevent internal bleeding;. Her blood level of vitamin C was only 0.06 mg per deciliter. When she was put on 1000 mg of vitamin C per day she regained normal health, qualified, however, by the surgery she had endured."

Without sufficient vitamin C, her blood vessels grew weak and leaked blood into her abdomen.

With sufficient vitamin C, her blood vessels grew stronger and stopped leaking.

Hmmmm. Hold that thought.

---------- ---------- ----------

Pauling and Rath looked at studies going back decades, and conducted research of their own. Their findings are in conflict with what we have been programmed to believe.

As naturopath and Pauling advocate/chronicler Owen R. Fonorow recalls on his website (**http://www.internetwks.com/owen/HeartCureR-D.htm**), "The theory that Cardiovascular Disease (CVD) is related to a deficiency of vitamin C was first proposed by the Canadian physician G. C. Willis in 1953. He found that atherosclerotic plaques form over vitamin-C-starved vascular tissues in both guinea pigs and human beings. In 1989, after the discoveries of the Lp(a) cholesterol molecule (*circa* 1964) and its lysine binding sites (*circa* 1987), Linus Pauling and his associate Matthias Rath formulated a unified theory of heart disease and invented a cure."

Willis was the first to suggest that heart arteries were damaged by high blood pressures within those arteries (much higher than the blood pressure in your arms) combined with mechanical stress caused by the constantly pounding heart beat.

Pauling and Rath studied Willis' observation that plaque does not form randomly throughout the body. For example, in a heart bypass, veins from the leg are used, partly because they contain no plaque.

There was also this curiosity to consider. Wouldn't you think, if plaque build-up were caused by cholesterol particles floating in the blood, that the tiniest blood vessels would be the first to plug up? Wouldn't large vessels hosting a torrent of blood, such as carotid arteries in the neck and coronary arteries, flush away those particles before they could build up, and wouldn't those vessels be the last to develop blockages? But the opposite is true.

Based on the work of Willis and others, Pauling and Rath concluded that arteries in human hearts are deprived of adequate vitamin C. The root cause of coronary artery disease, they determined, is artery weakness, "localized scurvy," brought on by lack of enough vitamin C reaching the heart.

In their weakened condition, coronary arteries yield to high pressures and a constantly pounding pulse. Lesions (shallow cracks) then develop.

"Why only humans and not other creatures?" the two wondered. Their answer is that almost all mammals, (except for guinea pigs, fruit bats, primate monkeys and humans) naturally produce their own vitamin C.

Most animals' bodies use enzymes to convert bloodsugar to the ascorbate form of vitamin C. It is continually produced in their livers. For example, it has been reported, a 160-pound goat creates in its body about 13,000 milligrams of vitamin C per day.

According to the online publication, Human Gene Therapy (**http://www.liebertonline.com/doi/abs/1 0.1089/hum.2008.0106**), genetic research is under way that may someday lead to humans regaining the ability to create their own vitamin C. Researchers in 2008 successfully restored the ability to do just that in a strain of lab mice that had been bred to no longer produce its own vitamin C. In less than 23 days, gene therapy was so effective that vitamin C levels in the defective mice were restored to those of normal mice who naturally make their own.

So, long term, perhaps we will make enough of our own vitamin C to ward off heart disease, stroke and other organ failure. Keeping our individual cells healthy, as Pauling and Rath suggest, just might be the Holy Grail of longevity, the real "Fountain of Youth."

For now, though, the solution Pauling and Rath hit upon to strengthen heart arteries was this: daily intake of massive doses of vitamin C.

---------   ----------   ----------

Meanwhile, Pauling and Rath wondered, suppose you do restore strength to heart arteries, then what do you do to clean out existing plaque formations?

That is when they turned their attention to the chemical make up of the gummy substance that builds up in weakened arteries. What was it, actually? And, why was it there?

Beginning during the Korean War, scientists began examining the artery walls of deceased GI's and of other people who died of coronary artery disease. They were looking for LDL, the "bad" form of cholesterol, and by golly, they found it. For decades it was settled science that plaque build-up in artery walls consisted mainly of LDL. But in the late 80's Dr. Rath, working with researchers U. Beisiegel, A. Niendorf, K. Wolf, and T. Reblin, pursued work begun by Berg and others, and began looking at another substance found in plaque. It was the sticky cousin of LDL, another form of lipoprotein identified as Lp(a).

Lp(a) is a highly-oxidized variety of LDL that attaches itself to a specific protein (Apo A). Together, they become Lipoprotein A or Lp(a). These really sticky molecules of Lp(a) seemed to be the glue in a process that patches arteries from the inside. It could also be implicated in how blood clots form.

---------- ---------- ----------

Pairing Pauling's decades of interest in vitamin C with Rath's work involving Lp(a) was a seminal event. Pauling brought the artery-healing theory of vitamin C therapy. With Rath came the idea that something other than LDL was plugging up heart arteries. That "something," he and his colleagues had concluded, was Lp(a).

Others, too, were studying Lp(a). As early as 1986 the American Heart Association's very own journal, *Circulation*, was reporting the findings of another group: They reported Lp(a) was associated with CAD (coronary artery disease) in women of <u>all</u> ages. It was a factor, too, in men younger than 55. The apparent threshold for coronary risk was Lp(a) concentrations of approximately 10 to 13 mg/dl. Lp(a) **appeared to be a major coronary risk factor** in the white patients studied, with a significance approaching that of the level of LDL or HDL cholesterol. *Circulation* 74, No. 4, 758-765, 1986. (Emphasis mine--DHL)

Drug companies remain unimpressed. They have continued to focus attention (yours, mine, and our doctors) on "bad" LDL and "good" HDL.

---------   ----------   ----------

But why were these plaque blockages forming in the first place, and what did they have to do with weakened arteries? Pauling and Rath set about finding out.

To make a long story short, they knew, from the research of others, that weakened arteries were likely to develop shallow cracks. "Lesions" is the term doctors use.

Picture a tubeless tire with a small puncture. The body's natural reaction is to send repairs to the site of the lesion. Like a blow-out patch on the inside of that tire, plaque builds up over a lesion to prevent an arterial blow-out. In other words, plaque is a *symptom* of heart disease, but not the cause.

Lp(a), Pauling and Rath concluded, was like a fireman rushing to the scene of a fire. Except, the body uses Lp(a) to patch up those lesions (shallow cracks) that develop in arteries weakened by a lack of sufficient vitamin C. Those sticky surfaces of Lp(a) plug the crack on one side. They then grab any passing LDL to help build a scab over the site of the wound.

So, perhaps rather than being a bad thing – to be compressed against artery walls with a balloon, or held in place with a stent, or removed with lasers or a type of "Roto-Rooter" – plaque is saving lives every day. Until, that is, it breaks loose or otherwise blocks a vital artery.

The twin goals, then, for Pauling and Rath, were to a) strengthen heart arteries with massive doses of vitamin C to prevent the need for the body to build up plaque, and b) to clear those restored arteries safely of existing plaque to prevent it from causing future heart attacks. They knew how to strengthen arteries. Now, what to do about that gummy plaque buildup?

---------   ----------   ----------

Coming back to Pauling's theory of using vitamin C to restore health to heart arteries, it is noteworthy that some heart specialists are now calling arthrosclerosis a "systemic disease." By that they mean it is necessary to treat all the heart's arteries, not just areas where plaque has built up.

In a New York Times article published March 21, 2004, a Dr. Waters of the University of California is quoted, talking about his 1999 research, "'We were saying that atherosclerosis is a systemic disease. It occurs throughout all the coronary arteries. If you fix one segment, a year later it will be another segment that pops and gives you a heart attack, so systemic therapy ... has the potential to do a lot more.''

Of course the "systemic therapy" Waters had in mind was even greater use of "statins or antiplatelet drugs." Has your doctor yet recommended them for your children?

--------- ---------- ----------

That Pauling and Rath were proposing vitamin C to strengthen arteries -- and proposing a course of action to remove plaque build up everywhere in the body -- was and remains medical heresy to this day.

Yet, it makes so much sense.

Have your gums ever bled when you flossed your teeth? Have you ever had a nosebleed for no apparent reason? Have you ever had a wound that was slow to heal? If so, you may have (had) a deficiency of vitamin C in your system.

Often -- it would appear from Pauling and Rath's work -- lack of vitamin C is overlooked when a person develops a chronic condition (which adds stress to the body and further depletes already inadequate ascorbate stores). Tell-tale symptoms of scurvy may appear but the correct diagnosis may be missed and instead called some chronic disease (i.e., poor wound healing in diabetics, hemorrhages in diseases like Crohn's and ulcerative colitis, etc.).

---------- ---------- ----------

My personal opinion?

Most of us are walking around suffering from what I would call *"lack-of-adequate-vitamin C disease,"* but our doctors – encouraged by the pharmaceutical industry – just keep treating our *symptoms*. More on this in Chapters Six and Seven.

CHAPTER FOUR --

Why the "Pauling Protocol" Works

(READER CAUTION: This is the technical stuff. Cinch up thinking caps NOW.)

Pauling was big on something called collagen

Now, in Hollywood, collagen injections are popular, mostly to inflate lips and to fill wrinkles, lines and scars on the face and sometimes the neck, back and chest. Collagen means, "glue producer" (kola = glue in Greek) – because glue has been made for centuries by boiling animal sinew and hooves. The gelatin in Jell-O comes from the collagen in cow or pig bones, hooves, and connective tissues.

But Pauling was focused on the collagen that forms, naturally, inside of you. In fact collagen is the most abundant protein in your body. It forms into fibers which are stronger than iron wire of comparable size. These fibers provide strength and stability to all body tissues, including your arteries.

And collagen formation requires large amounts of vitamin C.

Here is a transcript of poor old, doddering imbecile (as Big Pharma portrayed him) Linus Pauling from that YouTube video someone posted after his death (**http://www.youtube.com/watch?v=A5d-ba4DK0e4**). It was created just a few months before he died.

"Collagen is made in rather large amounts in human bodies and in the bodies of other mammals. It strengthens the blood vessels and the skin, and the muscles, and the bones, and the teeth. A very important substance. You can't make collagen without using up vitamin C. Collagen is made from another protein, 'procollagen,' by hydroxlilating Lys-ile and Pro-ile residues in the procollagen and converting them into hydroxi-Lys-Ile and hydroxi-Pro-Ile residues. With every hydroxyl group that is introduced, one ascorbate ion (one molecule of vitamin C) is used up. ... most animals manufacture their own vitamin C in their livers, and they manufacture it in such large amounts that their blood vessels and other tissues are stronger than those of human beings and do not develop the sort of lesions that result in overt cardiovascular disease such as humans get."

Oh, yes, obviously doddering and demented, wasn't he?

Expanding on that Pauling quote, collagen is the most abundant protein in the body. While literally a fiber, collagen acts like a "glue," one that holds our cells together. Collagen is actually the body's preferred repair substance -- for closing wounds, healing blood vessels, or helping the skin look its best.

The extremely tiny collagen fiber looks like a 3-strand rope. It contains a strand of L-glycine molecules, a strand of L-proline molecules, and a strand of L-lysine molecules. Under a powerful microscope, these strands can be seen twisted around each other. They do, in fact, look like a rope. When an injury happens and the collagen fiber breaks, the frayed ends dangle exactly like a damaged rope.

As Pauling explained in scientific language, above, if enough ascorbate (vitamin C) is available, the amino acid molecules at the broken ends are "hydroxylated." That means the "end" molecules of Lglycine, lysine and proline are chemically changed. They become L-hydroxyglycine, L-hydroxylysine and L-hydroxyproline.

This chemical process allows those frayed ends to be spliced back together (much like boatswain's mates who worked for me in the Navy used to splice rope). As Pauling explained, "With every hydroxyl group that is introduced, one ascorbate ion (one molecule of vitamin C) is used up." In other words, vitamin C is absolutely essential for the production and repair of collagen, *and vitamin C is destroyed during the process*. That is why consuming large amounts of vitamin C – to replace vitamin C destroyed in this process -- is key to healing damaged arteries.

As we saw in Chapters One and Three, the first part of the Pauling and Rath Protocol is consumption of massive amounts of vitamin C. The vitamin C nourishes collagen in our trillions of cells and restores health to damaged blood vessels. Because your body flushes it from your system so quickly, the only way to flood heart vessels with enough vitamin C to keep them healthy is to take large doses, preferably at least three times each day.

As for those three key amino acids, L-glycine is the least complex and, in general, the body always makes enough. L-lysine and L-proline, though, are not always in sufficient supply. So, in following the Pauling/Rath protocol, you need to take L- lysine and L-proline supplements, along with vitamin C, to ensure adequate collagen repair.

---------- ---------- ----------

While Pauling was interested in collagen and the health of heart arteries, Rath was looking at the nature of that "blowout patch," the build up of plaque inside weakened arteries. If arteries could be restored to health, how could the plaque be prevented from breaking loose, possibly to cause a fatal heart attack?

The answer was to remove the plaque; but how?

All lipoproteins are molecules made of proteins and fat. They carry cholesterol and other necessary substances through the blood. While nearly everyone else was looking at LDL and HDL, Rath and his colleagues had been studying Lp(a).

Lipoprotein (a) is a type of cholesterol carrier found *only* in species that *do not* produce their own vitamin C. When there is not enough vitamin C circulating in your arteries to keep you healthy, your body looks to Lp(a) to patch damaged blood vessels and keep you from dying of internal hemorrhage. So --surprising to most of us – LDL, on which the entire statin industry is based, is *not* the main culprit.

Sticky Lp(a) particles circulate in your blood. When a blood vessel wall is damaged, they are attracted to those frayed collagen "ropes" we talked about earlier. In particular, in the absence of an adequate supply of vitamin C, they bond with the lysine fragments.

As Lp(a) begins to coat your broken lysine strands, free lysine in the blood is drawn to the Lp(a). LDL is then attracted to the other two. This process continues as lysine, Lp(a) and LDL are drawn from your blood to build ever-larger amounts of plaque. Gradually this "blow out patch" grows in thickness. Over time, it can reduce the inner diameter of an artery and restrict its capacity to carry blood. In the worst case, you have a heart attack and die.

A report from Berkeley HeartLab, a wholly-owned subsidiary of Quest Diagnostics, finds the following about Lp(a): "Lipoprotein(a) was first described in 1963 and subsequently ascribed a role as a cardiovascular risk factor. Lp(a) is a plasma lipoprotein, produced in the liver, very similar in structure and density to LDL, having a cholesterol-rich triglyceride (TG) core encapsulated by a layer of phospholipids and free cholesterol. Like all non-high density lipoprotein (non-HDL) particles, every Lp(a) has a single molecule of apolipoprotein B (apoB) attached to the surface. Similar to LDL particles, both lipid core and attached apoB in Lp(a) are atherogenic."

(Author's comment: In layman's terms, atherogenic means "hardening of the arteries." And, just to clear up the "a" and "B" confusion, there is this from Wikipedia: "Lipoprotein(a) [Lp(a)] consists of an LDL-like particle and the specific apolipoprotein(a) [apo(a)], which is covalently bound to the apoB of the LDL like particle. Lp(a) plasma concentrations are highly heritable and mainly controlled by the apolipoprotein(a) gene [LPA] located on chromosome 6q26-27.")

I swear my eyes crossed while reading that.

---------- ---------- ----------

If you waded through all that, you figured out that Lp(a) is like LDL, *yet different*. And that difference is what Rath and Pauling were able to exploit.

They went looking for something that could circulate in the blood and both neutralize and remove Lp(a) after arteries had been restored to health by vitamin C. They found just that in L-Lyzine.

That's right. Not only does L-Lyzine play a role in repairing collagen and heart arteries, but molecules of this substance circulating in your blood are also able to bond with a receptor on the surface of the Lp(a) molecule – no longer needed for that "blow out patch" -- and gradually drag it away to the liver to be flushed from your system. The LDL scavenges waste products and returns with them to your liver also -- to the same liver that then sends out fresh HDL, packed with nutrients for every cell in your body.

---------- ---------- ----------

Later, Rath and Pauling found that L-Proline is equal to, or even better than L-Lyzine in its ability to remove Lp(a). L-proline is a unique amino acid. It prefers to be in oil rather than water. L-proline is thus lipophilic as opposed to L-lysine, which prefers water and is hydrophilic (not to be confused with my great uncle, who was an alcophilic. But I digress).

Lp(a) is a combination of a water-loving protein (apo a) and oily cholesterol. Pauling and Rath theorized that lipophilic L-proline would block receptors on the oily portion of Lp(a). When they added L-proline to their vitamin C and L-lysine solution, the effects were astounding. Blockages completely disappeared. That's what happened to me.

---------- ---------- ----------

So, here's the deal in a nutshell. Vitamin C is sacrificed to repair your dangling lysine and proline strands of collagen. This process prevents and/or repairs artery damage. When there is abundant vitamin C available – and with your artery health restored -- there are no longer any frayed lysine and proline strands in vessel walls. There is no longer a "fit" for Lp(a)'s receptor sites. Gradually, Lp(a) particles (or plaque patches) start to erode from the now-healthy artery walls.

Massive doses of vitamin C promote healthy heart arteries. Large doses of L-Lyzine and L-Proline clean up the mess left behind (arterial plaque), and sweep the arteries clean. Maintenance levels of these three over-the-counter, inexpensive supplements can keep things that way.

Reference those photos of my own arteries on the cover and throughout this book.

---------- ---------- ----------

To add further emphasis to the vitamin C and Lyzine theory, there is this. Pauling and Rath were granted yet another U.S. patent (# 5230996). You can find it displayed here: **http://www.internetwks. com/pauling/lpatent2.html**. It was for a solution containing vitamin C and L-lysine, this one *to remove plaques from donor organs* prior to transplant surgery. (emphasis mine--DHL)

When a transplanted organ is in place, blood must quickly disperse through the new organ or its tissue will quickly die. Bathing transplanted organs in this vitamin C-lysine solution before implantation *removed plaques in major vessels* and greatly improved transplantation outcomes. Pretty impressive for vitamin C and a lowly amino acid, don't you think?

Afterthought: Oh, how I wish I had paid better attention in high school science and biology classes. I might have been able to bore you with even greater details on how all this works.

Tossing a bone to the scientists among us …

Vitamin C Chemical Structure

Source: About.com Chemistry http://chemistry.about.com/od/ factsstructures/ig/Chemic- al-Structures---V/Vitamin-C--- Ascorbic-Acid.htm

L-Lysine Chemical Structure:

Source: About.com Chemistry (http://chemistry.about.com/od/imagesclipartstr uctures/ig/Amino-Acid-Structures/Lysine.htm)

L-Proline Chemical Structure:

Source: About.com Chemistry
http://chemistry.about.com/od/fact
sstructures/ig/Chemical-Struc-
tures---P/L-Proline.-eXf.htm

"OH-NOooo" **Source: Mr. Bill**

CHAPTER FIVE

What Pauling and others have suggested adding to the Protocol

Remember … Pauling and Rath's "Unified Theory" borrows from the naturopathy branch of medicine -- unlike its opposite, Big Pharma's "Lipid Theory," which treats diseases and symptoms with patentable synthetic chemicals, like statin drugs.

And remember, too, Pauling was focused on restoring health to each of the trillions of individual living cells that make up your body. He reasoned you can not do that – in most instances – simply with chemicals and drugs.

Throughout the ages and up until the early 1900's, our bodies depended on natural substances for their health. All wild animals still do. Wild animals don't get injections. They don't pop pills. Mostly, they are able to get all the nutrition they need to remain healthy from the food they eat.

But have you looked at the food labels in you cupboards and refrigerator lately? "Natural" is not us. More and more, our systems are bathed by the foods we consume in preservatives, flavor enhancers and other unnatural substances to "improve" their taste and shelf life.

We get more salt in a bowl of soup than we need in an entire day. Essential vitamins and minerals are cooked out of processed foods. Worries are mounting that the beef, pork and poultry we consume are tainted with growth enhancers. It has even been suggested that little girls are coming of age sooner these days due to growth hormones in the meat they eat.

There is growing concern, too, that antibiotics given to animals raised for food are causing the viruses that attack us to mutate. Doctors and scientists are increasingly reporting new versions of some viruses that are less responsive to antibiotics for people.

In short, cells in every part of our bodies are under siege every day from many of the foods we eat and from chemicals older generations never experienced. While vitamin C is essential to the collagen that we need for healthy cells -- to coin a phrase --

man cannot live on ascorbic acid alone. We can no longer simply rely on our diet for the remaining nutrition our bodies require.

Realizing this, Pauling added to his three basic heart ingredients – massive doses of vitamin C, L-Lysine and L-Proline – a list of other vitamins and minerals he *recommends* for healthy bones, muscles, brains and teeth.

Following is a summary of Pauling's earlier recommended supplementation from his 1986 book, How to Liver Longer and Feel Better, as that list appears on the Cancer Survival website (**www.cancersurvival.com/help_pauling.html**)

> 1. Take vitamin C every day, 6 grams (g) to 18 g (6,000 to 18,00 milligrams [mg]) or more. Do not miss a single day.
>
> 2. Take vitamin E every day, 400 IU, 800 IU, or 1600 IU.
>
> 3. Take one or more Super-B tablets every day, to provide good amounts of the B vitamins.
>
> 4. Take a 25,000 IU vitamin A or a 15 mg, beta-carotene tablet every day.
>
> 5. Take a mineral supplement every day, such as one tablet of the Bronson Vitamin-Mineral Formula.

6. Keep your intake of ordinary sugar (sucrose, raw sugar, brown sugar, honey) to 50 pounds per year, which is half the present US average. Do not add sugar to tea or coffee. Do not eat high-sugar foods. Avoid sweet desserts. Do not drink soft drinks.

7. Except for avoiding sugar, eat what you like-but not too much of any one food. Eggs and meat are good foods. Also, you should eat some vegetables and fruits. Do not eat so much food as to become obese.

8. Drink plenty of water every day.

9. Keep active; take some exercise. Do not at any time exert yourself physically to an extent far beyond what you are accustomed to.

10. Drink alcoholic beverages only in moderation.

11. DO NOT SMOKE CIGARETTES.

12. Avoid stress. Work at a job that you like. Be happy with your family.

--------- --------- ---------

Nutritionist and health consultant Jonathan Campbell (**http://www.cqs.com/index.html**), in his 2005 booklet entitled "The End of Cardiovascular Disease," updated Pauling's 1986 list by suggesting the following supplements for good health.

Recommended Supplement	Recovery Mode	Maintenance Mode
Magnesium glycinate (or other magnesium-amino acid chelate)	Calcium 1,000 mg Magnesium 500 mg twice daily	Calcium 500 mg Magnesium 250 mg twice daily
Acetyl-L-Carnitine	500 mg. twice daily	500 mg. twice daily
Vitamin E	400 IU daily	400 IU daily
Beta carotene (vitamin A source)	20,000 IU daily in two doses	20,000 IU daily in two doses
Omega-3 (n-3) fatty acids	Pharmaceutical Grade Fish Oil 2000 mg EPA/1000 mg DHA daily	Pharmaceutical Grade Fish Oil 2000 mg EPA/1000 mg DHA daily
Coenzyme Q10	50-100 mg 3 times daily with meals	50-100 mg 3 times daily with meals
Methylsulfonylmethane (MSM)	1,000 mg twice daily	1,000 mg twice daily

N-acetyl-cysteine	500 mg twice daily	500 mg twice daily
Zinc	40-50 mg total	30 mg daily
Potassium Citrate	500 mg three times daily	500 mg three times daily
High-dosage Multi-Vitamin/Mineral Complex	Daily	Daily
Grapeseed Extract	150-300 mg daily	150-300 mg daily
Alpha Lipoic Acid	500 mg twice daily	500 mg twice daily
Chlorella	2,500 mg three times daily	2,500 mg three times daily
Lecithin granules	2 tblspns daily	2 tblspns daily
Organic Flaxseed Oil	2 tblspns daily	2 tblspns daily
Water	2 Quarts daily	2 Quarts daily
Soy Protein Drink	1/2 Scoop X3	1/2 Scoop X3
Copper	2 mg daily	2 mg daily

Others, too, have expanded on Pauling's list of suggested supplements for a healthy heart and body. For example, Thomas E. Levy, MD, JD (**http://tomlevymd.com/index.html**), in his book, *Stop America's #1 Killer*, recommends the following:

Recommended Supplement	Daily Intake
L-arginine	500 to 1,500 mg daily
Menatetrenone (vitamin K2)	3 to 9 mg daily
Cholecalciferol (vitamin D3)	400 to 1,000 IU daily
L-carnosine	200 to 1,000 mg daily
Thiamine (vitamin B1)	50 to 500 mg daily
Pyridoxine (vitamin B6)	25 to 100 mg daily
Riboflavin (vitamin B2)	5 to 15 mg daily
Pantothenic acid (vitamin B5)	10 to 15 mg daily
Biotin (vitamin B7)	300 to 500 micrograms daily
Folic acid (vitamin B9)	400 to 500 micrograms daily
Cobalamin (vitamin B12)	15 to 20 micrograms daily
Niacin (vitamin B3)	20 to 25 mg daily
Superoxide dismutase (SOD)	100 to 400 mg daily
Chondroitin sulfate C (chondroitin 6-sulfate)	500 to 1,500 mg daily
Glutathione	500 to 1,500 mg daily
Chromium	100 to 200 micrograms daily
Manganese	'0.5 to 1.0 mg daily
Selenium	100 to 200 micrograms daily
Vanadium	10 to 50 micrograms daily
Indium	25 to 50 micrograms daily
Boron	15 to 20 micrograms daily

The good news is several of the items in the above lists can be found in a good quality adult multi-vitamin. Most of the others are readily available.

BOTTOM LINE: Beyond vitamin C, L-Lysine, L-Proline, plus the basic list recommended by Linus Pauling, my personal recommendation is that you research according to your own needs. The above discussion is presented simply to make you aware that many others are continuing to add to the work of Pauling and Rath.

CHAPTER SIX

But What About Cholesterol? And What Do I Eat Now?

"Why do you think an egg yolk is full of cholesterol? Because it takes a lot of choles-terol to build a healthy chicken. It also takes a hell of a lot to build and maintain a healthy human being.

"In fact, cholesterol is so vital that almost all cells can manufacture cholesterol; one of the key functions of the liver is to synthesize cholesterol. It's vital for the proper functioning of the brain and it's the building block for most sex hormones."--Malcolm Kendrick, MD (MbChB MRCGP) peer-reviewer for the British Medical Journal, and member of The International Network of Cholesterol Skeptics (Thincs), quoted from his 2007 article, "Have we been conned about cholesterol?" published in the U.K. Daily Mail On Line.
http://www.dailymail.co.uk/health/article430682/H ave-conned-cholesterol.html)

Back a generation or two, it used to be really something when you heard "the rabbit died." Depending on the circumstances, it could mean great joy. At other times, women could become hysterical. Grown men cried. A dead rabbit meant some woman was pregnant.

Animal testing was the norm back then, and rabbits were perhaps more guinea pigs than Guinea Pigs. So it wasn't surprising, in 1956, when some bozos in white lab coats in South Africa force fed massive quantities of cholesterol to bunnies and then reported a large number of the poor little rabbits died.

Here is part of the cover page of their report, available on the Internet: (**http://onlinelibrary.wiley.com/doi/10.1111/j.1365-2141.1957.tb05535.x/abstract**):

Brit. J. Haemat., 1957, 3, 366.

Blood Coagulation Abnormalities Produced by Feeding Cholesterol to Rabbits

C. MERSKEY

Department of Medicine,* University of Cape Town, South Africa

ABNORMALITIES of blood coagulation have been observed in cholesterol-fed rabbits (Merskey, Sapeika, Uys and Bronte-Stewart, 1956). Rabbits which received cholesterol and phenindione (phenylindanedione, P.I.D., Dindevan) were noted to have a higher mortality (mainly from haemorrhage) than rabbits fed cholesterol without phenindione. Even without phenindione, rabbits receiving cholesterol developed a prolonged coagulation time and excessive amounts of residual prothrombin remained in the serum after coagulation. In general this defect developed as the serum cholesterol rose and there was correlation between elevation of the serum cholesterol and the development of the coagulation defect. In this paper the fully-developed coagulation abnormalities of the cholesterol-fed rabbits are described.

There you have it. Rabbits – which produce their own vitamin C and seldom develop heart disease – got saturated with gooey, sticky cholesterol that their bodies had no use for, and their arteries clogged up. When the cholesterol diet was withdrawn, the surviving bunnies had miraculous recoveries. The conclusion of this brilliant study? Cholesterol kills *people*. And, presto! A new fake "disease" was invented, and the race was on to find a so-called "cure."

That questionable beginning launched the "Lipid Theory" of heart disease. It speculates that harmful levels of a waxy substance (cholesterol) circulate in your blood. You need the "good" kind (HDL), but the "bad" kind (LDL) is just waiting for the opportunity to stick itself to otherwise healthy blood vessels and gum them up.

For some unexplained reason, LDL only does this in larger arteries (carotid, cardiovascular), where you might expect torrents of blood under high pressure would sweep it away. It seldom, if ever, blocks smaller arteries or veins. Go figure.

Here's the crash course. Your liver produces "lipoproteins" (i.e., lipids and proteins) which then circulate in your blood. Lipids are naturally occurring molecules that include fats; waxes; sterols; fat-soluble vitamins such as A, D, E and K; monoglycerides, diglycerides, and other substances.

Lipoproteins can be further defined as various types of cholesterol, triglycerides, fatty acids, and phospholipids, among others. There's an industry of folks who measure and quantify these things in your blood – and a much bigger, and very profitable, industry dedicated to manipulating their levels in your bloodstream.

In reality, your lipids are like military Meals Ready to Eat, carried by your blood stream to nourish cell membranes everywhere in your body. Everywhere. It's a closed loop, with HDL carrying fresh supplies to your cells, and LDL bringing waste products back to your liver.

Yet, the "Lipid Theory" tries to distinguish between "good" (HDL) and "bad" (LDL) cholesterol. It seeks to increase the former and diminish the latter.

Here's the problem. There is no evidence that the levels of these substances in your blood – or attempts at controlling them, for that matter – will increase (or decrease) your chances of dying from coronary artery disease.

One of my favorite people in the great cholesterol debate (see the quote from him that opened this chapter, plus his graph on the back cover of this book) is the Scottish M.D., Malcolm Kendrick, author of the book *The Great Cholesterol Con*. He's a favorite because he took the time to analyze a couple studies conducted by the World Health Organization (WHO).

In its global MONICA (Multinational MONItoring of trends and determinants in CArdiovascular disease) Project, WHO studied cholesterol levels in populations around the world. This was a major project, collecting decades of research by scientists in dozens of countries. The MONICA scientists also analyzed deaths by heart attack in a couple dozen countries. As luck would have it, fifteen countries or groups of people ended up in both reports.

Kendrick's approach was ingenious. He made a line graph of average cholesterol levels in those fifteen countries. Next he superimposed a second line graph over the first. This one, also from MONICA, studied "Death Rates from Heart Disease in Males Aged 35 – 74" *in those very same populations*.

Famously, lines from those two charts do not match. Not even close. Australian Aborigines have among the highest death rates from heart disease in the world. Yet, their cholesterol levels are by far the lowest among the fifteen regions studied. And Switzerland, with the highest blood cholesterol levels, has among the very lowest death rates from heart disease.

France, too, in what has become known as "the French Paradox" – because the French, whose delight in cheeses and creams is supposed to ramp up heart disease – have among the lowest heart death rates. Paradox, indeed.

There is a very short YouTube video of Dr. Kendrick with his graph. You can view it here: **http://www.youtube.com/watch?v=i8SSCNaaDcE&feature=player_embedded#**!

If it were not deadly serious, it would be funny, but here is a YouTube cartoon that adds perspective to Kendrick's work: **http://www.youtube.com/watch?v=GqdzJLOQM2I**

---------- ---------- ----------

So, besides (supposedly) gumming up arteries, what does cholesterol do for you?

Let's talk about your brain. It weighs about three pounds. Like much of your body, 78 percent of it is water. Protein accounts for about eight percent. Carbohydrates and other substances make up about 4 percent. Between 10 and 12 percent is fat (remember that the next time someone calls you a fathead; they'll be semi-correct). Much of that fat (gasp) is cholesterol.

Your brain is made up of several types of cells with specific functions. One kind seemed to do very little, and was pretty much ignored until 2001. Then, a group of German and French researchers discovered these cells weren't lazy after all. Called "glial cells," they contain cholesterol – in fact, they make their own cholesterol. What they do with it is the amazing part. They use the stuff *to encourage your brain to manufacture synapses.*

Synapses, you may know, are the junctions or pathways that enable one cell to communicate with other cells. They're existence makes it possible for you to think and remember. When those researchers put glial nerve cells in a Petri dish and added plain cholesterol, synapses began forming before their eyes (well, under their microscopes, actually, but you get the picture).

Dr. Duane Graveline, MD (**http://spacedoc.com/**), is a former flight surgeon for the U.S. Air Force. He conducted space medicine research, was a NASA astronaut, practiced as a family physician for 20 years, and wrote eight books during his retirement.

Yet, after six weeks on Lipitor, he experienced what is called "transient global amnesia" that lasted about six hours. During that time he could not remember most of his incredible life – nor recognize his wife and children. Concerned that Lipitor might have caused this, he stopped taking the drug despite his doctors' assurances.

A year later, when his doctors encouraged him to try Lipitor again, the amnesia soon returned, this time lasting 12 hours and sending him to the ER. Dr. Graveline's experiences led him to others who reported similar memory lapses after taking this drug. Further research resulted in his book, *Lipitor, Thief of Memory*.

In a subsequent book, *Statin Drugs Side Effects*, Dr. Graveline cites a study by Muldoon, et al that found "100% of patients placed on statins showed measurable decrease in cognitive function after six months, whereas 100% of placebo treated control patients showed measurable increase in cognitive function during the same time period."

---------- ---------- ----------

So, raise your hand if you want to deplete your brain of cholesterol. Didn't think so. But, you know, that may have already happened. That is, if you have ever taken statin drugs. Statins do not discriminate. They don't just diminish cholesterol levels in your blood. They rob vital cholesterol from every organ in your body -- including your brain.

I know this from personal experience. After all, I was on statin drugs a total of seventeen years. A few years ago I was so concerned about memory fog that I sought medical help. The good news was that my symptoms were not those of Alzheimer's. My IQ was still high, but my memory complaints were "inexplicable."

For instance, I cannot remember a string of numbers longer than about four or five digits. I enjoy watching NFL games on TV, but with few exceptions I cannot identify familiar faces of coaches and players on the sidelines. I enjoy watching the games, but if I step away from the TV I have difficulty remembering the score or most of the previous plays.

Similarly, I enjoy watching the post-game shows with my wife, who is an avid fan. I like the replays and the interviews. Yet, again with few exceptions, don't ask me who was interviewed after the show has ended.

This carries over to my writing.

I have been a professional writer most of my life – mostly press releases and short articles in various PR jobs (this is my first ever attempt at writing a book). I ran my own consulting business for medical practices, a company called "Patient Relations," for about six years.

So, I know how to write. Keeping a train of thought going, though, has become difficult. In working on a chapter like this one, for instance, I cannot tell you how many times I'll have to go back and read it from the beginning, so that I may gather my thoughts and continue.

Oddly, these lapses and losses of memory don't impact my ability to handle technical tasks. I can trouble shoot most computer glitches. Solutions come quickly to mind. I enjoy my Android smart phone, and have it loaded up with useful apps. Just don't ask me to name many of them without looking at the phone.

---------- ---------- ----------

Ever wonder who sets the target numbers for your HDL and LDL? Those numbers were adjusted downward again in 2004 – creating millions more patients who thus "need" statin drugs. More than a few eyebrows were raised at the composition of the panel behind the "**Third Report of the Expert Panel on Detection, Evaluation, and Treatment of High Blood Cholesterol in Adults (Adult Treatment Panel III)**."

Members of that board had more than a passing acquaintance with the companies that manufacture statin drugs, the same companies that stood to reap a fortune based on the panel's new numbers. Details about those relationships were revealed here:

"P III Update 2004: Financial Disclosure" (http://www.nhlbi.nih.gov/guidelines/cholesterol/ atp3upd04_disclose.htm)

"Dr. Grundy has received honoraria from Merck, Pfizer, Sankyo, Bayer, Merck/Schering-Plough, Kos, Abbott, Bristol-Myers Squibb, and AstraZeneca; he has received research grants from Merck, Abbott, and Glaxo Smith Kline."

"Dr. Cleeman has no financial relationships to disclose."

"Dr. Bairey Merz has received lecture honoraria from Pfizer, Merck, and Kos; she has served as a consultant for Pfizer, Bayer, and EHC (Merck); she has received unrestricted institutional grants for Continuing Medical Education from Pfizer, Procter & Gamble, Novartis, Wyeth, AstraZeneca, and Bristol-Myers Squibb Medical Imaging; she has received a research grant from Merck; she has stock in Boston Scientific, IVAX, Eli Lilly, Medtronic, Johnson & Johnson, SCIPIE Insurance, ATS Medical, and Biosite."

"Dr. Brewer has received honoraria from AstraZeneca, Pfizer, Lipid Sciences, Merck, Merck/Schering-Plough, Fournier, Tularik, Esperion, and Novartis; he has served as a consultant for AstraZeneca, Pfizer, Lipid Sciences, Merck, Merck/Schering-Plough, Fournier, Tularik, Sankyo, and Novartis."

"Dr. Clark has received honoraria for educational presentations from Abbott, AstraZeneca, Bristol-Myers Squibb, Merck, and Pfizer; he has received grant/research support from Abbott, AstraZeneca, Bristol-Myers Squibb, Merck, and Pfizer."

"Dr. Hunninghake has received honoraria for consulting and speakers bureau from AstraZeneca, Merck, Merck/Schering-Plough, and Pfizer, and for consulting from Kos; he has received research grants from AstraZeneca, Bristol-Myers Squibb, Kos, Merck, Merck/Schering-Plough, Novartis, and Pfizer."

"Dr. Pasternak has served as a speaker for Pfizer, Merck, Merck/Schering-Plough, Takeda, Kos, BMS-Sanofi, and Novartis; he has served as a consultant for Merck, Merck/Schering-Plough, Sanofi, Pfizer Health Solutions, Johnson & Johnson-Merck, and AstraZeneca."

"Dr. Smith has received institutional research support from Merck; he has stock in Medtronic and Johnson & Johnson."

"Dr. Stone has received honoraria for educational lectures from Abbott, AstraZeneca, Bristol-Myers Squibb, Kos, Merck, Merck/Schering-Plough, Novartis, Pfizer, Reliant, and Sankyo; he has served as a consultant for Abbott, Merck, Merck/Schering-Plough, Pfizer, and Reliant."

---------- ---------- ----------

At least half of those who have succumbed to coronary artery disease have had HDL and LDL numbers in the "normal" range. Rather than consider that they are on the wrong track, members of these panels consistently conclude we need a "new normal." Their numbers go lower – incidentally creating millions of new consumers for their pharmaceutical mentors – yet deaths from coronary artery disease remain stubbornly unaffected. Odd, isn't it?

---------- ---------- ----------

OK, so what does the Pauling/Rath diet consist of?

Pauling himself says to go back to a normal diet. Or, as Ben Franklin famously said, "All things in moderation."

If cholesterol is merely a boogey man, why play the no-cholesterol/low-cholesterol game? I have gone back to using real butter. I enjoy a flavorful, well-marbled steak from time to time. And deserts are no longer forbidden food (although, Pauling did warn us to cut our sugar consumption by half).

Am I gorging myself? Absolutely not. My wife has other health issues, so I am eating healthier with her. We consume a lot of salad, in part because we enjoy it. Portions on our plates are smaller, and more in line with dietary recommendations. Where we once enjoyed a porterhouse or sirloin, each, we now share halves of one. We switch around between beef, chicken and pork (I might eat more fish, but she dislikes it, nor will she cook it).

From all those years of "watching my cholesterol," I have to admit I've developed one or two acquired tastes. Much as I like saltine crackers, I can't stand the regular ones anymore. They taste greasy and lacklustre to me now, and I much prefer the fat-free kind.

After giving up milk decades ago, I resorted to rice and soy products, but none really pleased me. Then, a few years ago, a dietician suggested almond milk. I prefer it on my cereal now. Besides, I've read that cow's milk is designed to foster the growth of calves, and that no human over age six really needs that stuff.

But these are our personal peculiarities. The bottom line is, if you are following the Pauling/Rath protocol, enjoy what you want … in moderation.

---------   ----------   ----------

AND THIS JUST IN: "Researchers stopped a clinical trial when it failed to find any benefit from raising levels of HDL ('good') cholesterol with extended-release niacin. Adding the drug to a statin, a medication that lowers LDL ('bad') cholesterol, was expected to lead to a reduction in heart attacks and strokes. But there was no difference between those taking just a statin and people taking a statin plus niacin in how often heart disease developed. The study calls into question long-held beliefs about the benefits of raising levels of HDL cholesterol. But the findings may not apply to people with poorly controlled LDL or other risk factors for heart attack and stroke."-- Source: National Institutes of Health, May 26, 2011 (**http://www.nih.gov/news/health/may 2011/nhlbi-26.htm**).

Add to the above a Reuters report, "Low 'good' cholesterol doesn't cause heart attacks," (**http://www.reuters.com/article/2011/12/01/us-low-cholesterol-idUSTRE7B02S820111201**) referencing a study in the November 2011 Journal of Clinical Endocrinology and Metabolism.

Although a first glance analysis of data on nearly 70,000 people in Denmark seemed to show a link between low levels of high-density lipoprotein (HDL) -- the so-called "good" cholesterol -- and raised heart attack risk, there was a nagging problem. In people with a gene mutation that lowers HDL, heart attack risk was not found to be higher at all.

That finding suggests something other than low HDL must be causing heart attacks. Or, as Reuters reported, "'Association itself doesn't mean causality,' said lead author Dr. Ruth Frikke-Schmidt, a consultant in the Department of Clinical Biochemistry at Rigshospitalet in Copenhagen."

The results suggest that just having low HDL is not what raises the likelihood of a heart attack. "It's a total relook at what we thought was gospel," Dr. Christopher Cannon, professor of medicine at Harvard Medical School and editor of the American College of Cardiology's website, told Reuters.

CHAPTER SEVEN

How Come Drugs Seem to "Cure" Only SYMPTOMS?

At a press conference on July 2, 1992, Linus Pauling and Matthias Rath, MD presented their advances in vitamin research and the possible eradication of heart disease to the world. The pharmaceutical companies reacted immediately through the United States Food and Drug Administration (FDA). A nationwide campaign was started to prohibit all health claims in relation to vitamins and other natural substances.

Author's Disclosure: I received government pay checks for 24 years as a U.S. Navy officer (active and reserve) and in the decade of the 1970's (as environmental spokesman for the state of Maine). I started several businesses that did not survive long term. Yet I remain an unabashed advocate for free enterprise. The profit motive is what made the United States prosper.

That being said, when it comes to our health there is a cloud over the issue of decisions based on profits. In the past, the impact was thought to be felt mostly by those with "orphan diseases" (defined in the U.S. as illnesses with a prevalence of fewer than 200,000 individuals at any given time), which lacked research dollars mostly for lack of profit potential.

As I write this, however, new reports place us all at risk. Critical shortages have developed in drugs used in operating rooms as well as at local pharmacies. The situation is serious enough that some patients have died. The U.S. Food and Drug Administration now maintains a website, "Current Drug Shortages" (**http://www.fda.gov/Drugs/DrugSafety /Drug Shortages/ucm050792.htm**). It also offers a second website, **https://public.govdelivery.com/ accounts/USFDA/subscriber/new?topic_id=USFD A_22**, where you can subscribe so that you will be alerted if drugs you take are on the shortage list.

Why is this happening? The Institute for Safe Medication Practices, the American Society for Health System Pharmacists (ASHP), the American Society of Clinical Oncology (ASCO), the American Society of Anaesthesiologists (ASA) and the American Hospital Association (AHA) are studying the causes. In one of its papers, though, the Institute for Safe Medication Practices has called for "More effective FDA oversight, a comprehensive early warning system, and patient safety **and outcomes placed ahead of anyone's profit margins** ..." (emphasis mine)

Without profits, there would be no private sector pharmaceutical industry. But trouble arises when our traditional profit motive seems to guide decisions that run counter to the reality of our health care needs. I don't pretend to have a solution.

---------- ---------- ----------

Have you noticed the money Big Pharma makes peddling cures that often only treat symptoms? U.S. based companies alone brought in an estimated $307 billion globally in 2010, according to a 2011 pharmaceutical industry profile by IMS Health (**http://www.imshealth.com/portal/site/ims/menu-item.5ad1c081663fdf9b41d84b903208c22a/?vgnext-oid=fbc65890d33ee210VgnVCM10000071812ca2R-CRD**) in conjunction with PhRMA, (Pharmaceutical Research and Manufacturers of America, Washington, DC, **www.phrma.org**). That's just U.S. based companies.

Has it ever crossed your mind how much money those pharmaceutical companies stand to lose should a major disease actually be cured? How many have been eradicated in your lifetime?

OK, in my long lifetime I have to concede, we pretty much wiped out polio, yellow fever, malaria, mumps and other childhood diseases. But most of those were long ago.

Granted, there's been progress, especially in the treatment of many forms of cancer. Lives have been extended. Some blood born cancers have been "cured," but the best most patients can say about their particular cancer is it is "in remission." Often, too, the cures have been based on radical surgeries, removing breasts, lungs, lymph glands and other affected organs. AIDS has been brought under control – by a trade off, to a lifetime of enslavement to expensive drugs.

I'm not saying there is one, but just "what if" someone has already come up with an honest solution for a disease that plagues us? Like cancer, or Alzheimer's, or diabetes? Perhaps a cure based on vitamins and minerals, and not on chemical drugs?

Would Big Pharma, the AMA, the AHA and FDA welcome it with open arms, knowing it would wipe out billions in profits? Not if what they have appeared to do to promote statin drugs and diminish the Pauling/Rath cure for coronary artery disease is any example.

A big reason they continue to diminish Dr. Rath, as they did Pauling, is his outspoken, unequivocal criticism of Big Pharma. One example is his website, "What You Need to Know About the Fraudulent Nature of the Pharmaceutical Investment Business With Disease" (**http://www4.dr-rath foundation.org /open_letters/pharma_laws_history.html**).

---------- ---------- ----------

Linus Pauling had already experienced Big Pharma's backlash several years prior to his and Dr. Rath's heart cure announcement. As mentioned in Chapter 2, Pauling and a Dr. Cameron demonstrated that terminal cancer patients lived many years longer on massive doses of vitamin C alone than did others who received the recommended standard chemotherapy. You can read about their ordeal on the website "Natural Cancer Treatments" (**http://www.cancertutor.com/WarBetween/War_Pa uling.html**).

---------- ---------- ----------

"Dollars for Docs -- How Industry Dollars Reach Your Doctors"
Some have calculated that the pharmaceutical industry spends twice the amount of money it expends on research in its efforts to manipulate public opinion. Besides the large sums they spend on media advertising campaigns, to convince you to "ask

your doctor" about their latest, greatest patented miracle, Big Pharma apparently spends millions directly to influence doctors.

An article in the September 7, 2011, Orlando Sentinel, headlined, "Florida doctors taking millions of dollars in Big Pharma money," (**http://articles.orlan dosentinel.com/2011-09-07/health/os-doctors-phar ma-list-20110907_1_drug-companies-research-com panies-florida-doctors**) puts some local faces on the doctor influencing efforts of the pharmaceutical companies:

"Among those who were paid the most in Central Florida's five counties are Dr. Cxxxx Cxxxx, an Orlando researcher who received $918,938 from three drug companies; Jxxx Hxxx, a registered nurse in The Villages who was paid $111,295 by Eli Lilly; and Dr. Dxxxx Txxxxx, an endocrinologist at Florida Hospital Celebration Health who earned $67,509 from Lilly." (Author's note: the newspaper reveals their full names, so I don't feel compelled to do so here.)

"While some payments, such as those that support research, are necessary," the paper notes, "money paid to doctors to curry favor and encourage them to promote a company's medications crosses an ethical line, say industry watchdogs."

Beginning in 2013, federal law will require all drug and medical-device companies to disclose the amount and purpose of payments they give providers. Meanwhile, you can get a partial glimpse at what your doctor and/or others in your area have received.

ProPublica, the "website for journalism in the public interest," has created a tool based on data already released by a dozen pharmaceutical giants – representing roughly 40 percent of the U.S. drug market. Go to **http://projects.propublica.org/docdollars/** and enter your doctor's name, or just click on your state, then click "Search."

If similar profits could be made by peddling vitamins, do you suppose Big Pharma might be promoting vitamin therapy with equal gusto?

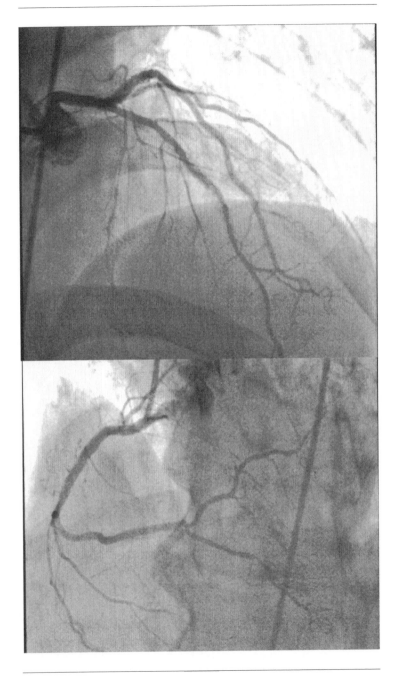

CHAPTER EIGHT

Why What You Don't Know About Statin Drugs Could
a) Cripple You, or
b) Wreck Your Brain or
c) Kill You

"The Netherlands Radar TV Survey of Statin Side Effects: '50,000 people were recently invited by e-mail to take part in an on-line survey by Radar Television in the Netherlands.

'27,692 replied. Of these, 4738 (17.1%) were on Statins. Of the 4738, 27.1% reported side effects. Theyhad a choice of: muscle pain, joint pain, digestion problems, loss of memory or other.
'748 (39.8%) reported muscle pain
'592 (31.5%) reported joint pain
'301 (16.0%) reported digestion problems

'239 (12.7%) reported loss of memory
'420 reported other effects.

"To me this is perhaps as close as we have ever come to the true incidence of statin drugs side effects and it is very alarming. We know the usual breakdown of side effects - 40% cognitive, 40% muscle and 20 % all the rest but this is the first survey as to incidence that I feel I can believe."
--*Duane Graveline, MD, MPH*
(http://www.spacedoc.com/ netherlands_radar_ survey.html)

"LIPITOR is not for everyone. It is not for those with liver problems. And it is not for women who are nursing, pregnant or may become pregnant. If you take LIPITOR, tell your doctor if you feel any new muscle pain or weakness. This could be a sign of rare but serious muscle side effects. Tell your doctor about all medications you take. This may help avoid serious drug interactions. Your doctor should do blood tests to check your liver function before and during treatment and may adjust your dose. Common side effects are diarrhea, upset stomach, muscle and joint pain, and changes in some blood tests." — *the official Lipitor disclaimer*

What's a little "muscle and joint pain," compared to preventing heart attacks, you might wonder. The phrase is repeated so blithely at the end of TV commercials for statin drugs that it might go unnoticed. Unless, that is, you have experienced it first hand.

In my 17 years of taking statin drugs, the pattern kept repeating. After anywhere from six to eighteen months, I would develop a dull ache. For me, it was always in the same spot, just beneath the lowest rib on my right side. It would gradually increase from that dull ache to a stabbing pain. "It can't be the statin," my doctors would say, "but let's take you off of it and see what happens." After a few days off the drug, invariably my pain would go away.

As luck would have it, another newly patented synthetic statin drug would have recently come on the market at that point – reflecting the constant need of the industry to stay a step ahead of patent expirations, when generic mimics of the original drug flood the market and drive down prices. My then-heart doctor would start me on this latest "miracle," and the pattern would be repeated.

Until, that is, we got to Lipitor. I thought I had finally found my simpatico statin. I was two-and-a half years into Lipitor, thinking all was fine. One night, talking with my cousin, a former nursing home employee, I said my hips had been aching a lot lately. Her immediate response was, "Are you taking Lipitor?"

At her urging, I went to see my new heart doctor a few days later. I asked him whether my aching hips could be related to the statin. "Let's find out," he said. "Stop taking it and let's see what happens."

What happened next shocked me. While the hip pain subsided, I suddenly developed excruciating pain in the big muscles of both legs. It got so painful that one day when I went to a Home Depot store I had to grab a shopping carriage in the parking lot just to keep myself upright. At the back of the store the pain became so intense I did not know whether I was going to make it back to my car. I believe what I experienced was a form of statin drug withdrawal.

"It couldn't have been the Lipitor," my new heart doctor exclaimed. "Statins don't do that," said my family doctor. Oddly, though, my leg pains gradually subsided. They were completely gone six weeks after stopping Lipitor, and they have never come back

"This could be a sign of rare but serious muscle side effects," the TV statin spokesperson opines in that famous low-key monotone disclaimer we have all heard hundreds of times. Well, it turns out, those serious side effects have a name.

Rhabdomyolysis is the breakdown of muscle fibers resulting in the release of muscle fiber contents (myoglobin) into the bloodstream. Some of these are harmful to the kidneys and frequently result in kidney damage. Your doctor knows this, and now you know why he or she sends you twice yearly for blood tests if you are on a statin drug. They are monitoring the drug's effects on your kidneys.

---------- ---------- ----------

In Chapter Six we discussed the important role cholesterol plays in your brain. It is vital to the formation of new synapses, the channels that connect individual cells and make it possible for you to think. I described the permanent damage to my own cognitive processes that I attribute to 17 years on statin drugs. We also learned from Dr. Graveline's book, **Statin Drugs Side Effects**, of a study that found "100% of patients placed on statins showed measurable decrease in cognitive function after six months, whereas 100% of placebo treated control patients showed measurable increase in cognitive function during the same time period."

---------- ---------- ----------

If a doctor has you on a statin drug, but has not told you to take the supplement Coenzyme Q10 (or CoQ10), he or she might be setting you up for memory issues, or even premature death, either from a heart attack or other organ failure.

CoQ10 is a key factor in energy transfer inside your body's individual living cells. Statin drugs block cholesterol production through something called the "mevalonate pathway." Unfortunately, cholesterol is not the only traveler along this pathway. It shares the space with CoQ10, among other things.

So, when statins block this pathway, they also hinder the body's uptake of CoQ10. Not only that, our bodies' ability to synthesize CoQ10 begins decreasing after age 21. For most of us over age 50, the only way to maintain an adequate level of CoQ10 is through over-the-counter supplements. Few of us bother, making the potential impact from the blocking function of statin drugs all that much worse.

Ironically, doctors put us on statins to protect our heart arteries. Yet, the heart is usually the first organ to be affected by low levels of CoQ10. That's because the heart requires the most energy of any bodily organ to keep working. What appears to be cardio- myopathy or congestive heart failure might actually be the result of too little CoQ10. But you won't see CoQ10 deficiency on a death certificate.

---------   ----------   ----------

We've met him elsewhere in this book, but now is a good time to talk about another hero of mine in this conflict. He is "SpaceDoc" (**www.SpaceDoc.com**), Duane Graveline, MD, MPH, Former USAF Flight Surgeon, Former NASA Astronaut, Retired Family Doctor. You can read his official biography here: **http://www.spacedoc.com/Graveline_bio.htm**.

Doctor Graveline's website is a veritable Who's Who of medical professionals and researchers who have come to distrust all the hype about statin drugs and their supposed benefits. Much of what I have learned on this topic has come from the work of this group of mavericks. I encourage you to explore SpaceDoc's website as well as his links to works by the others displayed on his home page.

For instance, Dr. Graveline's extensive report, "Statins and CoQ10 Deficiency," can be found here: **http://www.spacedoc.com/statins_CoQ10.htm**

Further Reading

Following is the suggested reading list quoted from the website for **The International Network of Cholesterol Skeptics** (THINCS) (**http://www.thincs. org/news.htm**)

John von Radowitz, (The Independent): **"85% of new drugs offer few benefits"** (**http://www.independent.co.uk/lifestyle/health-and-families/health-news/85-of-new-drugs-offer-few-benefits-2054972.html**)

Christopher Hudson (Telegraph): **"Wonder drug that stole my memory."** Statins have been hailed as a miracle cure for cholesterol, but little is known about their side effects. Read also the 140 comments that follow the article, but

beware, they are scary. (**http://www.telegraph ph.co.uk/health/4974840/Wonder-drug-that-stole-my-memory.html**)

Melinda Wenner Moyer (Scientific American): **"It's Not Dementia; It's Your Heart Medication."** Why cholesterol drugs might affect memory. (**http://www.scientificamerican.com /article.cfm?id=its-not-dementia-its-your-hear t-medication**)

Tom Naughton: **"Big Fat Fiasco: how the misguided fear of saturated fat created a nation of obese diabetics."** A humourous speech with a serious content. Five parts, on Youtube (**http://www.fathead-movie.com/inde x.php/2010/10/28/video-of-the-big-fat-fiasco-s peech/**)

Uffe Ravnskov*: *Ignore the Awkward! How the Cholesterol Myths are Kept Alive.* (**http://www.amazon.com/Ignore-Awkward-Cholesterol-Myths-Alive/dp/1453759409/ref=s r_1_ 1?ie=UTF8&s= books&qid=1288080387& sr=1-1**)
A new book.about how prominent scientists have turned white into black by ignoring all conflicting observations; by twisting and exaggerating trivial findings; by citing studies with opposing results in a way to make them look supportive; and by ignoring or scorning the work of critical scientists. Includes a short and simplified version of his previous book

Denise Minger: **The China Study: Fact or Fallacy**. Is this book, authored by Colin Campbell, really "one of the most important books about nutrition ever written," as stated on the cover by Dean Ornish? It is rather one of the most misleading! Read this review! (**http://rawfood sos.com/2010/07/07/the-ch-ina-study-fact-or-fallac/**)

David H. Freeman: **"Lies, Damned Lies and Medical Science."** The Atlantic Nov. 2010 (**http://www.theatlantic.com/magazine/print/2010/11/lies-damned-lies-and-medical-science/8269/**)

PublicCitizen, Dec 16, 2010: **"Rapidly Increasing Criminal and Civil Monetary Penalties Against the Pharmaceutical Industry: 1991 to 2010"** (**http://www.citizen.org/hrg1924**)

Malcolm Kendrick*: **"The Cholesterol Myth Ex posed."** A short Youtube presentation (**http://www.youtube.com/watch?v=i8SSCNaaDcE**)

Lipitor Paradox. A funny but also sad Youtube movie (**http://www.youtube.com/watch?v=G qdz JLOQM2I**)

Emily Deans: **"Low Cholesterol and Suicide."** Psychology Today 21 March 2011 (**http://www.ps ychologytoday.com/blog/evolutionary-psychiatry/201103/low-choles-terol-and-suicide**)

Dwight D Lundell*: **"The Cholesterol Scam."** A view from an experienced thoracic surgeon. (**http://www.spacedoc.com/statin_scam**)

Stephanie Seneff*: **"How Statins Really Work Explains Why They Don't Really Work."** **(http://people.csail.mit.edu/seneff/why_statins_ dont_really_work.html**)

* Authors who are members of THINCS are marked with an asterisk.

CHAPTER NINE

Women and Statin Drugs

"To date, no large trial of women statin users who already have cardiovascular disease has been shown to increase life expectancy by one day. More importantly, the use of statins in women at lower risk has not increased life expectancy nor prevented heart attacks and stroke.

"It raises the question whether women should be prescribed statins at all. I believe that the answer is no. Statins fail to provide any overall health benefit in women.

"The more recent heart protection study was hailed as a success for men and women, but despite the hype there was no effect on mortality in women."

--The Great Cholesterol Con by Malcolm Kendrick; John Blake Publishing (http://www.amazon.com/dp/1844546101? tag=spacedoc20&camp=14573&creative=327641&li nkCode=as1&creativeASIN=1844546101&adid=0A 4G2X0R82EAQEJZ4QDF&&refreURL=http%3A %2F%2Fwww.spacedoc.com %2Fgreat_cholesterol_con)

"In a smaller group of women — those who already have heart disease — the data suggests that statins can reduce heart-related deaths. But as Dr. Beatrice Golomb, a professor of medicine at the University of California, San Diego, says, they don't reduce deaths overall. '**Any reduction in death from heart disease seen in the data has been completely offset by deaths from other causes,**' she says. Which raises the question: If statins do not help prolong women's lives, why are so many women taking them?" — **Time Magazine**, March 29, 2010 (http://www.time.com/time/magazine/article/0,9171 ,1973295,00.html#ixzz1YKfbXl2Y)

"For women with heart disease, using statin drugs reduces the chance they'll have a heart attack. But for some women—those who only have elevated

LDL (or 'bad' cholesterol levels) with a very low risk for cardiovascular disease — the benefit of statins should be weighed against the potential harm from taking them." **-- Consumer Reports**, June 2010 (**http://www.consumerreports.org/health/best-buy-drugs/drug-safety/statins-inwomen/overview/index.htm**)

Not being a woman myself, I have no personal testimony to add here, except this:

High doses of Vitamin C, L-Lysine and L-Proline never hurt anyone. If you are a woman, start your own research thread with a Google search for "Statins and women."--The Author

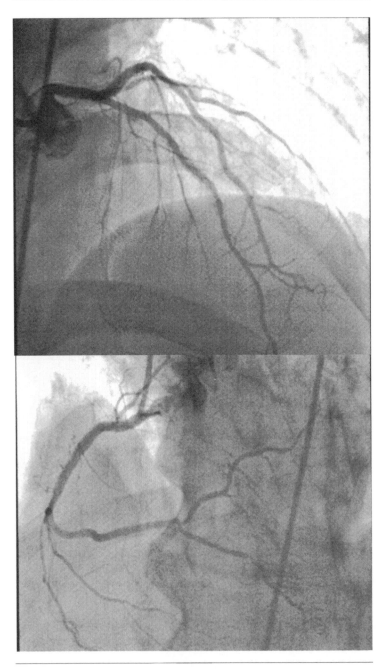

CHAPTER TEN

If Your Doctor Says "Don't Try This," Find Another Doctor

"Any physician, or panel of hospital-based physicians, claiming that vitamin C is experimental, unapproved, and/or posing unwarranted risks to the health of the patient, is really only demonstrating a complete and total ignorance or denial of the scientific literature. A serious question as to what the real motivations might be in the withholding of such a therapy then arises..... ignorance of medical fact is ultimately no sound defence for a doctor withholding valid treatment, especially when that information can be easily accessed." – Thomas E. Levy, M.D., J.D. http://www.whale.to/a/vitc45.html (**Read Dr. Levy's latest book on Vitamin C,** *Primal Panacea,* now available)

My first cardiologist treated me from age 48 to 63. He implanted those three stents in my heart in September, 2003. In January 2004 he issued the letter of "permanent limitation" you see displayed right after the Introduction of this book.

A year later, his group of physicians elected to no longer accept the insurance plan I had at that time. Disappointed, I was left with no choice but to find a new heart doctor, so I don't know how he might have reacted to my vitamin C regimen. I have not seen him since.

I've been with my "new" cardiologist for the last seven years. When I eventually developed serious side effects from Lipitor – as I'd had with all the other available statins – he was stumped. There were no statin alternatives remaining to try.

When I brought him the results of my Internet research – the Pauling/Rath patented cure for heart disease – he was skeptical yet open minded. He agreed to work with me to monitor my condition. This included checkups, ordering fasting blood tests, and occasional stress tests. I had to agree to continue taking four other prescription medications plus low-dose aspirin, but I am now down to just Plavix (which he advises I should always take because of those stents) and low-dose aspirin.

My family doctor, too, has been supportive. I think he has been skeptical, but he has never said so to my face. He, too, has monitored my condition, and he was dually impressed with the results of my July 2011 angiography. He agreed, seeing those photos of my heart's x-rays (on the cover and throughout this book), and reading the cardiac interventionist's report, my coronary artery disease is gone.

So my advice to you is this. There are a growing number of cardiologists and family doctors who have heard about the Pauling/Rath Protocol, and an increasing number who are open minded enough to work with patients who want to try it. How far that openness extends may depend, in part, on how well your body has responded to his or her preferred treatment with statin drugs. Remember, I had actually run out of statin options.

The point is, if, having read this book and after conducting your own additional research, you want to pursue the Pauling/Rath protocol, there are doctors out there who will work with you. Don't be afraid to interview several until you find the right fit. And, above all, don't go it alone. Remember the old adage; he who treats himself has a fool for a doctor.

Start by discussing this with your current doctor(s). If you are met with resistance, start interviewing replacements.

APPENDIX A

My Actual Daily Intake, and Why I Take All Those Pills

It probably helped that I grew up in a home where my mother was an ardent reader of Prevention Magazine. She took several vitamins, and she started me on a children's multi-vitamin at an early age. I don't think she obsessed about them, but that magazine had lots of articles about the benefits of vitamins for this or that human condition. Let's just say my childhood experience made me open minded on the subject of vitamins and minerals.

I was in my forties, though, before I took much more than an adult one-a-day type of multi-vitamin. At some point, I began on my own – but always with my doctors' awareness -- to expand into what some might consider more naturopathic uses of vitamins and minerals to promote wellness and prevent illness.

At any rate, let's look at what's on my supplement menu for today ... and why.

HEART
Vitamin C, 6,000 mg daily, divided in three equal doses. This is my maintenance dosage; for the first couple months I took 10,000 mg. See Chapters One and Four for details.

L-Lyzine, 3,000 mg daily, divided in three equal doses, to cleanse Lp(a) plaques from heart arteries. See Chapters One and Four for details.

L-Proline, 3000 mg, divided in three equal doses, also to prevent Lp(a) build up. See Chapters One and Four for details.

L-Arginine, 500 mg, one tablet daily in the AM for heart health. Recommended by Dr. Levy. See Chapters Five for details.

Plavix, 75 mg, once daily in the AM. My current heart doctor has advised me to stay on this prescription platelet thinner because of those three annoying stents that were placed in my heart's arteries in 2003. He says stents occasionally fray, their loose pieces then sticking out into the blood stream.

There, they have been known to collect enough sticky platelets to either a) block an artery and cause a heart attack, or b) send a blood clot to the brain or lungs. So, I'll probably have this souvenir medication from my former coronary artery disease with me – along with those stents – for the rest of my life.

Fish Oil, morning and night, for its Omega-3 Fatty Acids which support heart health and also reduce blood clotting. There is a prescription version, Lovaza (with a little synthetic tweaking, of course, to make it patentable and expensive). However, for a lot less money you can buy high-grade fish oil over the counter. I try to stay with enteric coated capsules; they help prevent fishy aftertaste. Here are a couple websites discussing Lovaza versus over-the-counter fish oil:

http://www.trackyourplaque.com/blog/2008/12/lovaza-rip-off.html

http://vintagefemail.blogspot.com/2008/05/lovaza-.html

Aspirin, 81 mg, single dose at night. This is another blood thinner and, again, stent related. If you have no stents, ask your doctor before taking aspirin. It can lead to stomach bleeding.

CoQ10, 150 mg, single dose in the AM. If you are still on statin drugs, this is a MUST. I continue to take it to strengthen heart muscle and to counter the damage to heart and brain cells done over the 17 years I was on statin drugs.

BRAIN/NERVOUS SYSTEM

My greatest concern regarding my years on statin drugs has more to do with my head than my heart. If you have read Chapter Eight, you know about my memory issues. If you have not read the book by Duane Graveline, MD, *Lipitor, Thief of Memory*, or visited his website, **www.SpaceDoc.com**, I hope you will do both without delay. That goes double if you are taking any form of statins.

Bacopa Extract, 225 mg tablets or capsules, two in the morning and two at night. Bacopa is important in traditional Ayurvedic medicine. It has been used, particularly in India, for several thousand years. Recent studies have indicated it can aid memory and promote a sense of well-being. This is new to my regimen.

Quoting from the E-Scripts Drug Digest (**http://www.drugdigest.org**), "In India, several small studies have evaluated the effectiveness and safety of bacopa for children as young as six years old. Generally, children given about 1,000 mg (one gram) per day of bacopa had improvements in memory, observation, and reaction time. None of the children had side effects.

"In another study, children with attention deficit hyperactivity disorder (ADHD) took 50 mg of bacopa or a placebo (identical but inactive medications) twice a day for 12 weeks. The children who took bacopa showed general improvements in learning and memory."

Could Bacopa be the gentle alternative to Ritalin?

As for myself, I do think it is helping. There was no "aha!" moment, but there's been a gradual release from the tension of trying to come up with the right word in conversation. I guess you could say I feel more confident, more relaxed, and I seem to be able to remember little things better. Like short shopping lists, or placing more names with faces of actors on TV shows or movies. Some days are better than others, but over all I believe it has helped. Or is it all in my mind? Hah!

CoQ10, (see HEART section, above). Statin drugs deprive the brain and other organs of this needed substance. Quoting Wikipedia, "This oil-soluble, vitamin-like substance is present in most eukaryotic cells, primarily in the mitochondria. It is a component of the electron transport chain and participates in aerobic cellular respiration, generating energy in the form of ATP. **Ninety-five percent of the human body's energy is generated this way**. Therefore, those organs with the highest energy requirements —such as the heart, liver and kidney —have the highest CoQ10 concentrations." (Emphasis mine – author)

Vitamin B12, 1,000 mcg, once daily in the AM, to promote homocysteine for health of nervous system.

STOMACH
Omeprazole (generic Prilosec), prescribed by my MD to control Gastro-Intestinal Distress (GURD). I

have had this condition for many years, going back long before I began the Pauling/Rath protocol.

Folic Acid, 800 mcg, once daily, to boost pancreatic health/insulin production.

Probiotic Supplement, one capsule daily in the AM. Recommended by a nutritionist to keep "good" bacteria flourishing in my gut. I purchase the Sustenex brand for its promise to survive passage through stomach acids and deliver a greater quantity of healthy bacteria to colonize my small intestine.

Vitamin B6, 50 mg, one tablet daily in the AM., to boost pancreatic health/insulin production.

JOINT HEALTH
Glucosamine/Chondroitin, 1500 mg/1200 mg, respectively; one tablet in am and one at night. I have been taking this for several years and it seems to be working. As I approach age 70, I can still deep knee bend, stand and walk without pain.

BONE HEALTH
Magnesium w/Chelated Zinc, 400 mg/15 mg, one tablet morning and night.

MUSCLE HEALTH
Potassium Gluconate, 99 mg, one tablet daily in AM to prevent muscle cramping. I began taking this to ward off side effects of statin drugs, and have continued it to preserve muscle tone.

VISION

Lutein, 20 mg, one capsule every morning, on the recommendation of my ophthalmologist.

Vision Formula vitamin capsule ("eQuate" Brand from Wal-Mart), 1 tablet daily every morning. When my ophthalmologist warned several years ago that I had the beginning signs of cataracts, I heard Paul Harvey touting the benefits of an expensive brand of vision vitamin formula. He said it could prevent or reverse cataracts, among other benefits. I discovered the less expensive brand at Wal-Mart was nearly identical to the expensive version. So I started taking this in addition to the Lutein the eye doctor had recommended. At my last checkup I mentioned she has never again brought up the subject of early cataracts. "That's because nothing has changed," she replied.

SENIOR HEALTH

"Mature Adult Multi-Vitamin," one tablet daily in the morning. Linus Pauling recommended this. I take it in addition to my other vitamins and supplements because it might fill in items I would not get otherwise. Remember that figure from earlier, that on average there is one admission per year to American emergency rooms for anything vitamin related, but 700,000 Americans each year go to the ER for emergencies due to prescription medications.

Vitamin B150 Complex, once daily in the AM. This supplement contains 150% or more of the FDA recommended daily allowance of all the B vitamins. Remember, the "daily allowance" is FDA's best guess at the *minimum* amount of a particular vitamin or supplement our bodies need. That is how they concluded we need only 60 mg of vitamin C each day, versus the 6,000 mg or more in the Pauling/Rath protocol. I take this complex to complement my other sources of the B vitamins.

ANTI-AGING

Resveratrol, 500 mg, one capsule daily at noon. This ingredient found in red wine was touted a few years ago by Barbara Walters, Dr. Oz and others because in laboratories it extended the lives of mice and lesser life forms. Perhaps it can do the same for humans. Time will tell (wry wit intended).

[Urgent: See the discussion in Appendix B, regarding attempts by Big Pharma to corner the Resveratrol market, too.]

ALLERGIES

Guaifenesin, 400 mg, "as needed" for mucous relief. It is the key ingredient of literally dozens of over-the-counter products. My allergist prescribed it, but I haven't needed it much since I started on weekly allergy shots in March 2011 (only about four years of allergy shots remaining as of this writing, but they do seem to help). My allergies include most grasses, dust, mold, cats, etc. (our cat – a stray Iadopted against my wife's and my own better judgment -- is not allowed in the bedroom).

ANTIOXIDENT
Selenium, 200 mcg, one tablet daily in the AM. Of course, Vitamin C and other supplements I am taking serve secondarily as antioxidants, too.

Vitamin E, 600 iu, once daily in the AM. It has also been demonstrated to support cardio, prostate and overall health. If you have heard that this vitamin is "controversial," visit this website: **http://www.leaflady.org/E_controversy.htm**.

IMMUNE SYSTEM
Vitamin D3, 400 iu, one tablet daily in the AM, supports the immune system and overall health. Of course, doctors will tell you, vitamin D is also important for bone health in the young and the old. Our bodies actually make vitamin D when exposed to the sun.

PROSTATE HEALTH
Bee Pollen, 550 mg, one capsule morning and night. Thirty or more years ago, I read about Swedish research indicating that Bee Pollen and Zinc together delay or prevent enlargement of the male prostate gland. I have been taking them ever since. Only time will tell whether it works, but blood tests to date indicate no signs of prostate cancer. Is my urine flow that of a young man? Uh, no. Golden flow is not a part of the Golden Years for us guys.

Zinc, 50 mg, one tablet in the AM (see above).

Saw Palmetto, 450 mg, two capsules morning and night.

WEIGHT CONTROL (reduction of belly fat)
Chromium Picolinate, 800 mcg, one tablet daily

That's the sum of stuff I take on a daily basis. Whether and how much those other than the BIG THREE (Vitamin C, L-Lyzine, L-Proline) had any role in reversing my coronary artery disease is hard to say.

Remember, this is the collection of vitamins and supplements I have chosen for myself. I have taken many of them for years (before and subsequent to my coronary artery disease). I am not recommending them, and I am not a medical doctor.

Each of us is a unique individual, with unique needs. You and your doctor should decide what is best for you.

APPENDIX B

Will You Let the U.S. Government Take Away Your Vitamins and Supplements?

<u>Orthomolecular Medicine News Service,</u> January 19, 2010 (http://orthomolecular. org/resources/omns/v06n04.shtml): **"There was not even one death caused by a dietary supplement in 2008, according to the most recent information collected by the U.S. National Poison Data System. The new 174-page annual report of the American Association of Poison Control Centers, published in the journal Clinical Toxicol-**

ogy, shows zero deaths from multiple vitamins; zero deaths from any of the B vitamins; zero deaths from vitamins A, C, D, or
E; and zero deaths from any other vitamin.

"Additionally, there were no deaths what-
soever from any amino acid or herbal
product. This means no deaths at all from
blue cohosh, echinacea, ginkgo biloba, gin-
seng, kava kava, St. John's wort, valerian,
yohimbe, Asian medicines, ayurvedic
medicines, or any other botanical. There
were zero deaths from creatine, blue-green
algae, glucosamine, chondroitin, melaton-
in, or any homeopathic remedies.

"Furthermore, there were zero deaths in
2008 from any dietary mineral supplement.
This means there were no fatalities from
calcium, magnesium, chromium, zinc, col-
loidal silver, selenium, iron, or multiminer-
al supplements. Two children died as a result of medical use of the antacid sodium bi-
carbonate. The other "Electrolyte and Mineral" category death was due to a man acci-
dentally drinking sodium hydroxide, a
highly toxic degreaser and drain-opener.
"No man, woman or child died from nutritional supplements. Period."

In Chapter Three we discussed how Big Pharma, together with the AMA and FDA, almost drove all naturopaths out of the medical practice. Thanks to organizations like Prevention, and later the advent of the Internet, vitamin and mineral producers and practitioners have survived and rebounded.

And yet, American emergency rooms only see, on average, <u>one patient per year</u> with an adverse reaction to vitamins and minerals. They see an average 700,000 per year due to pharmaceutical side effects and/or overdoses (**http://www.cdc.gov/Medication Safety/ program_focus_activities.html**).

<u>**None of that can explain this:**</u>
Just as I was putting the finishing touches on this book, I was made aware of efforts to thwart our access to these non-prescription products. The back story is pretty ugly. Long held patents are running out on the block buster cash cows of Big Pharma, and profits stand to plummet. If they can create synthetic (and thereby patentable) versions of the stuff we get now over the counter -- and at the same time deny access or drive prices of the natural versions out of sight -- their good times can continue . . . at our expense.

One example is Resveratrol. This ingredient found in red wine was touted a few years ago by Barbara Walters, Dr. Oz and others because it may have anti-aging properties. One U.S. manufacturer, a small company called Sirtris, was purchased for

$720 million in 2008 by GlaxoSmithKline. Where-upon, according to an article in the New York Times (**http://www.nytimes.com/2011/01/11/science/11agi ng.html**), the giant company cancelled clinical trials.

Among reasons the Times pointed to was this: "In addition, from a commercial point of view, Res-veratrol is a natural substance and not patentable." GSM bought Sirtis, the Times opined, because its re-search facilities might be able to create a synthetic (and thereby patentable) version.

Direct acquisition of all the vitamin and supplement manufacturers, though, would cost Big Pharma a bundle – not to mention the bad publicity. But sup-pose … with a little help from their friends in Con-gress, and their lackeys in the U.S. Food & Drug Ad-ministration … they might drive prices of vitamins and supplements sky high?

Little manufacturers would fall by the wayside. Big Pharma could pick up the slack, charging prescrip-tion prices or, even better, gaining prescription status for synthetic knock offs of the real things.

Read about their latest attempt, the "Dietary Supple-ment Labeling Act of 2011" (S. 1310), sponsored by Senator Richard Durbin (D-IL), here: **http://www.f-dalawblog.net/fda_law_blog_hyman_phelps/2011/ 07/legislation-introduced-to-improve-dietary-sup-plement-safety-bill-would-significantl y-increase-burden.html**

Writer and Critical Care Nurse Byron J. Richards, has been chronicling the efforts of Durbin and the FDA:

- "FDA Propaganda Attempts to Destroy the Dietary Supplement Industry," 8-23-11 (**http://www.newswithviews.com/Richards/byron213.htm**)
- "FDA's Scheme to Reclassify Nutrients as Drugs," 8-3-11 (**http://www.newswithviews.com/Richards/byron211.htm**)
- "Senator Durbin and the FDA Viciously Attack Dietary Supplements," 7-26-11 (**http://www.newswithviews.com/Richards/byron210.htm**)

Your help is needed. Visit Operation Push Back here: **http://operationpushback.com/**.

Another easy way for you to take action and communicate your position to your two Senators is on the new website, PopVox: **https://www.popvox.com/bills/us/112/s1310**.

To date, this piece of legislation has only attracted one single co-sponsor. Stay alert, though, and let your members of Congress know where you stand on this issue.

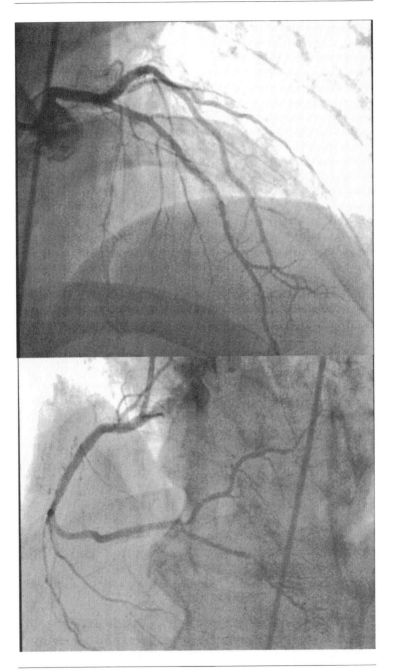

APPENDIX C
References and Credits

CHAPTER ONE – The End
- U.S. Patent # 5278189
(http://patft.uspto.gov/netacgi/nph-Parser?
Sect1=PTO1&Sect2=HITOFF&d=PALL&p=1&u=
%2Fnetahtml%2FPTO
%2Fsrchnum.htm&r=1&f=G&l=50&s1=5278189.P
N.&OS=PN/5278189&RS=PN/5278189)
– filed in 1994 by American scientist Linus Pauling
and German doctor Matthias Rath, MD, and titled
"Prevention and treatment of occlusive cardiovascular disease with ascorbate and substances that inhibit the binding of lipoprotein (A)"

CHAPTER TWO – Was Linus Pauling Nuts?
- Wikipedia, **"Linus Carl Pauling"** (**http://en-
.wikipedia.org/wiki/Linus_Pauling**)
- Book: **Vitamin C and the Common Cold**
[Paperback] by Linus Pauling
(**http://www.amazon.com/Vitamin-Com-
mon-Cold-Linus-
Pauling/dp/0425064557/ref=sr_1_1? ie=UTF
8&qid= 1326504309&sr=8-1**)

CHAPTER THREE – What did Pauling and Rath learn about Heart Disease?

* Book, *How to Live Longer and Feel Better* [Hardcover and Paperback] by Linus Pauling (Original 1986 Edition: **http://www.amazon.com**
* **/How-Live-Longer-Feel-Better/dp/0380702894**)

  (20th Anniv. Update, May 1, 2006: **http://www.amazon.com/How-Live-Longer-Feel-Better/dp/0870710966/ref=sr_1_fkmr0_2? s=books&ie=UTF8&qid=1326577073&sr=1-2-fkmr0**)

* Book: *Vitamin C and the Common Cold* [Paperback] by Linus Pauling (**http://www.amazon.-com/Vitamin-Common-Cold-Linus-Pauling/dp/0425064557/ref=sr_1_1? ie=UTF 8&qid= 1326504309&sr=8-1**)

* **Website, Orthomolecular.org: (http://www.or-thomolecular.org/index.shtml)**

* **Wikipedia, "Scurvy" (http://en.wikipedia.org/wiki/Scurvy)**

* Naturopath and Pauling advocate/chronicler **Owen R. Fonorow website: (http://www.inter-netwks.com/owen/HeartCureRD.htm)**

* **Paper: Lipoprotein (a) in the arterial wall** -- U. Beisiegel, A. Niendorf, K. Wolf, T. Reblin and M. Rath. European Heart Journal (1990) 11 (Suppl. E),   174-183   (**http://www4.dr-rath-foundationorg /THE_FOUNDATION/About_Dr_Matthias_Ra th/publications/pub03.htm**

- **AHA Publication: Circulation 74, No. 4, 758-765, 1986,** "Association of levels of lipoprotein Lp(a), plasma lipids, and other lipoproteins with coronary artery disease documented by angiography (in PDF Format")
(**http://www.google.com/url?
sa=t&rct=j&q=&esrc=s&source=web&cd=1&s
qi=2&ved=0CCEQFjAA&url=http%3A%2F
%2Fcirc.ahajournals.org%2Fcontent
%2F74%2F4%2F758.full.pdf&ei=Fd0QT7T-
fL4WFtgeqtvGRAg&usg=AFQjCNGIp-
kbP7sdYOZXGq-mGi29seSDjDA&sig2=fCZb3
AvheD8alKUd6bF8Sg**

- **New York Times article,** "New Heart Studies Question the Value Of Opening Arteries," published March 21, 2004
(**http://www.nytimes.com/2004/03/21/us/new-
heart-studies-question-the-value-of-open-
ing-arteries.html?pagewanted=4**)

- **Website:** COMPARING THE "LIPID THEORY" WITH THE "UNIFIED THEORY"
(**http://www.ourhealthcoop.com/pdf/MikeCi-
ell_unified_theory.pdf**)

CHAPTER FOUR – Why the "Pauling Protocol" Works

- **YouTube Video:** "Vitamin C, Heart Disease, Cancer, Collagen, Linus Pauling" (**http://www.y-
outube.com/watch?v=A5dba4DK0e4**)

- **Website:** COMPARING THE "LIPID THEORY" WITH THE "UNIFIED THEORY" (**http://www.ourhealthcoop.com/pdf/MikeCi-ell_unified_theory.pdf**)
- **Berkeley HeartLab report:** "Lipoprotein(a) [Lp(a)]" (**http://www.bhlinc.com/cirm-print.php? chapter=16**
- **U.S. patent # 5230996,** "treatment prior to trans-plantation" (**http://www.internetwks.com/pauli ng/lpatent2.html**)
- **About.com:** Chemistry, Chemical Structure of L-Lysine (**http://chemistry.about.com/od/im-agesclipartstructures/ig/Amino-Acid-Struc-tures/Lysine.htm**)
- **About.com:** Chemistry, Chemical Structure of L-Proline (**http://chemistry.about.com/od/facts-structures/ig/Chemical-Structures---P/L-Pro-line.-eXf.htm**

CHAPTER FIVE – What Pauling and others have suggested adding to the Protocol

- Pauling's recommended supplementation as of 1986, from the website Cancer Survival (**http://www.cancersurvival.com/help_paul-ing.html**)
- Jonathan Campbell website: (**http://www.cqs.com/index.html**)
- Thomas E. Levy, MD, JD website: (**http://www.tomlevymd.com/**)

- Owen R. Fonorow, Orthomolecular Naturopath, website: (http://www.internetwks.com/owen/bio.htm)
- Book: Thomas E. Levy, MD, JD, **Stop America's #1 Killer** (http://www.amazon.com/Stop-Americas-Killer-Thomas-Levy/dp/0977952010)

CHAPTER SIX – But What About Cholesterol?

- Malcolm Kendrick, MD (MbChB MRCGP), 2007 article, **"Have we been conned about cholesterol?"** U.K. Daily Mail On Line (**http://www.dailymail.co.uk/health/article-430682/Have-conned-cholesterol.html**)

- Report: **"Blood Coagulation Abnormalities Produced by Feeding Cholesterol to Rabbits"** (**http://onlinelibrary.wiley.com/doi/10.1111/j.1365-2141.1957.tb05535.x/abstract**)

- Book: *The Great Cholesterol Con*, Malcolm Kendrick M.D. (**http://www.amazon.com/Great-Cholesterol-Really-Causes-Disease/dp/1844543609**)

- YouTube video: Dr. Kendrick with his graph comparing cholesterol levels in specific populations against deaths from heart disease in those same countries (**http://www.youtube.com/watch?v=i8SSCNaaDcE&feature=player_embedded#**)

- Spoof cartoon supporting Dr. Kendrick's work (**http://www.youtube.com/watch?v=GqdzJLOQM2I**)

- Books: *Lipitor, Thief of Memory*.and, *Statin Drugs Side Effects*, Duane Graveline, M.D., MPH (**www.SpaceDoc.com**)

- **"Third Report of the Expert Panel on Detection, Evaluation, and Treatment of High Blood Cholesterol in Adults (Adult Treatment Panel III)."** (http://www.nhlbi.nih.gov/guidelines/cholesterol/)

- **National Institutes of Health ATP III Update 2004: Financial Disclosure** (reveals financial connections of those setting cholesterol target levels with the companies that manufacture andsell cholesterol drugs) **(http://www.nhlbi.nih.gov/guidelines/cholesterol/atp3upd04_disclose.htm)**

CHAPTER SEVEN – How Come Drugs Seem to "Cure" Only SYMPTOMS?

- Website, **"The Rath/Pauling Manifesto"**: **(http://www4.dr-rathfoundation.org/PHARMA CEUTICAL_BUSINESS/The_Chemnitz_Progra mme/chemnitz11.htm)**

- U.S. Food and Drug Administration website, **"Current Drug Shortages" (http://www.f-da.gov/Drugs/DrugSafety/DrugShortages/ucm0 50792.htm)**

- Institute for Safe Medication Practices **paper on shortages of prescription drugs (http://search.ismp.org/cgi-bin/hits.pl?**

in=517791&fh=80&ph=1&tk=j-LQ%26%20-LQ
%26gp%20pWeL%3An% 26I%2

0pWeL%3An%26Igp%20LQ%26p%20pWeL
%3An%26Ip&su=cnPPKthhwww.Aq
%3FK.WEzh%26gwqIgPPgEqhcOePgOcEghcE-
PAOIgqh200 10321Y2.cqK&qy=gnep-
%20uIqeLg-A&pd=1)

- 2011 pharmaceutical industry profile **(2010 U.S. drug sales, published by imshealth.com – In PDF Format) (http://www.imshealth.com/deployedfiles/ims/Global/Content/Insights/IMS %20Institute%20for%20Healthcare%20Informatics/IHII_Use OfMed_report1_.pdf)**
- Web Site, **"What You Need to Know About the Fraudulent Nature of the Pharmaceutical Investment Business With Disease" (http://www4.dr-rath-foundation.org/open_lett ers/pharma_laws_history.html)**
- Web Site, **"Natural Cancer Treatments" (http://www.cancertutor.com/WarBetween/War _Pauling.html)**
- Orlando Sentinel article, **"Florida doctors taking millions of dollars in Big Pharma money," (http://articles.orlandosentinel.com/2011-09-07/health/os-doctors-pharma-list-20110907_1_ drug-companies-research-companies-florida-doctors)**
- ProPublica website, **"Dollars for Docs" (http://projects.propublica.org/docdollars/)**

CHAPTER EIGHT – Why What You Don't Know About Statin Drugs Could, a) Cripple You, or b) Wreck Your Brain or c) Kill You

- Website of Duane Graveline, MD, MPH, on the Netherlands study **(http://www.spacedoc.com/netherlands_radar_s urvey.html)**

- Lipitor Official Website (Scroll to bottom for **"Important Safety Information"**) (http://www.lipitor.com/)

- **Rhabdomyolysis explained** by PubMed Health **http://www.ncbi.nlm.nih.gov/pubmedhealth/P MH0001505**

- Dr. Graveline's books: *Statin Drugs Side Effects* **(http://www.space-doc.com/)** *Statin Damage to the Mevalonate Pathway,"* **(http://www.spacedoc.com/statin_damage_mev alonate.html)**

- Website for The International Network of Cholesterol Skeptics (THINCS) **(http://www.thinc-s.org/news.htm)**

CHAPTER NINE – Women and Statin Drugs
- Book: *The Great Cholesterol Con* by Malcolm Kendrick; **(http://www.amazon.com/Great-Cho-lesterol-Really-Causes-Disease/dp/184454 3609)**

- Time Magazine article, **"Do Statins Work Equally for Men and Women? (http://www.time.com/time/magazine/article/0,9171,1973295,00.html#ixzz1YKfbXl2Y)**

- Consumer Reports Magazine article, **"Women and statins: When the drugs may not make sense"** (http://www.consumerreports.org/health/best-buy-drugs/drug-safety/statins-inwomen/overview/index.htm)

CHAPTER TEN – If Your Doctor Says "Don't Try This," Find Another Doctor

- *"Vitamin C And The Law, A Personal Viewpoint"* by Thomas E. Levy, M.D., J.D. **(http://www.whale.to/a/vitc45.html)** "This article may be reprinted free of charge provided 1) that there is clear attribution to the Orthomolecular Medicine News Service, and 2) that both the OMNS free subscription link **http://orthomolecular.org/subscribe.html**

    and also the OMNS archive link **http://orthomolecular.org/resources/omns/index.shtml** are included.

ADDENDUM A – My actual daily intake, and why I take all those pills

- Website, Orthomolecular.org article, **"No** Deaths from Vitamins, Minerals, Amino Acids

or Herbs"
(**http://orthomolecular.org/resources/omns/v06n 04.shtml**) "This article may be reprinted free of charge provided 1) that there is clear attribution to the Orthomolecular Medicine News Service, and 2) that both the OMNS free subscription link **http://orthomolecular.org/subscribe.html**

and also the OMNS archive link **http://ortho-molecular.org/resources/omns/index.shtml**
are included.

- Website, Medical Knowledge Base **("MedKB"), "Drug Errors Send 700,000 to ER Every Year"** (**http://www.medkb.com/Uwe/Forum.aspx/al-ternative/21414/Drug-Errors-Send-700-000-to-ER-Every-Year**)

- **E-Scripts Drug Digest** (**http://www.drugdi-gest.org**)
- Book, *Prostate Disorders and Natural Medicine*, **By Rita Elkins** (**http://www.rawpower.com/Books/Ailments/B ook-Prostate-Disorders-and-Natural-Medicine-0185.html**)

Websites Studied in Researching this Book (Not in any particular order)
- **The Cure for Heart Disease: Condensed** By Owen R. Fonorow, Copyright 2004 (**http://www.internetwks.com/owen/Heart-CureRD.htm**)

- Pauling-Therapy, **"The Cause and Non-prescription Cure for America's #1 Killer"** (http://paulingtherapy.com/)
- Internetworks Website (**http://www.internetwks.com/pauling/index.html**)
- **Excerpt of Chapter 7** from the book, *Practicing Medicine Without a License,* by Owen Fonorow (PDF Format) (http://www.practicingmedicine-withoutalicense.com/protocol/)
- Pauling video on the body's ability to absorb vitamin C (**http://www.youtube.com/watch?v=QXiUcU3rz3s**)
- Pauling video, "Cure for Heart Disease...Without Drugs or Surgery"

  (**http://www.youtube.com/watch?v=-GRUIiYlziw&NR=1**
- **Linus Pauling Pt 2 (**BBC Heretics of Science Series - 1994**) Vitamin C**

  (**http://www.youtube.com/watch?v=s99_L4LAds**)
- **Vitamin C, Heart Disease, Cancer, Collagen, Linus Pauling**

  (**http://www.youtube.com/watch?v=A5d-ba4DK0e4**)
- Pauling on his research with Rath (**http://www.youtube.com/watch?v=-sfn2mUwf4&feature=related**)
- NYT article, **"New Heart Studies Question the Value Of Opening Arteries"** (http://www.nytimes.com/2004/03/21/us/new-

heart-studies-question-the-value-of-opening-arteries.html?pagewanted=4&src=pm)

- "Lipoprotein (a) in the arterial wall," U. Beisiegel, A. Niendorf, K. Wolf, T. Reblin and M. Rath, European Heart Journal (1990) 11 (SUPPL. E), 174-183 (http://www4.dr-rath-foundation.org/THE_FOUNDATION/About_ Dr_Matthias_Rath/publications/pub03.htm)
- Restoring the Human Body's Ability To Make Vitamin C (http://www.lewrockwell.com/sardi/sardi91.html)

Additional Resources

- The Linus Pauling Institute: Micronutrient Information Center.

  (http://lpi.oregonstate.edu/infocenter/vitamins/vitaminC/index.html)

- Our Health Co-op - Heart Plus: Vitamin C, L-Lysine & L-Proline (http://nexwell.net/eshop/inx_detail.asp?tcPageKind=detail&tcModeCode=1287)

- Orthomolecular Medicine News Service (OMNS)

  (http://www.orthomolecular.org/resources/omns/index.shtml)

- **Vitamin C And The Law -- A Personal Viewpoint** by Thomas E. Levy, M.D., J.D. (**http://www.whale.to/a/vitc45.html**)

- Dr. Levy's Website (**http://www.tomlevymd.com/**)

- Vitamin C Foundation's Videos of Pauling and others (http://www.vitamincfoundation.org/videos/)

- **Vitamin C Saves Dying Man** (Note the dozens of reference links at the bottom) (**http://open.salon.com/blog/jeffrey_dach_md/2010/10/20/vitamin_c_saves_dyingman_by_jeffrey_dach_md**)

- **IF YOU HAVE RECENTLY HEARD THAT VITAMINS ARE SUPPOSEDLY HARMFUL,** you may want to read "**How to Make People Believe Any Anti-Vitamin Scare . . . It Just Takes Lots of Pharmaceutical Industry Cash**" (**http://www.doctoryourself.com/safety.html**)

About those two photos on the cover and repeated throughout this book:

Both images are X-rays of my heart's arteries, taken during an exploratory angiogram conducted at Florida Hospital Orlando on July 27, 2011. I turned 70 years old in January 2012. Nurses in the "cath lab" said they hoped their own arteries right then looked as good as mine. The interventional cardiology specialist who performed the procedure proclaimed my heart healthy (*"free of obstructive disease,"* were his written words) as did my family doctor, based on the cardiologist's report.

The upper photo is of my Left Anterior Descending (LAD) artery bundle, commonly known to heart doctors as "the widow maker." At one point, it contained a blockage of 85 percent. Later, my heart became home to three metal mesh stents. The only damage this cardiologist could now find involved those stents.

The lower photo displays the clean arteries on the back side of my heart. That straight line is actually the X-ray image of the catheter that was inserted through my thigh, into my femoral artery and then threaded into my heart. Through it, contrasting dye was injected that would then light up the X-rays. Dark spots are intersections, where a branch attaches to the main vessel. They are dark because we are looking into the trunk of a wide open vessel, so the camera picks up a greater amount of dye in the blood passing through that point.

My change in heart health occurred *after* 17 years of bad reactions to every statin drug (Lipitor was the last and the worst). It was only after I had run out of statin options that I turned in desperation to searching the Internet. That's how I discovered the 1994 patent that changed my life. It might change yours, and that's what this book is about.

(For Information about the facing photographs, see preceding page)

About the graph on the <u>Back</u> Cover.

Americans typically describe cholesterol levels in milligrams per deciliter, commonly expressed as mg/dl. In other parts of the world and among scientists, the measure often used is millimoles per litre (MMOL/L). The factor to calculate between the two is **38.7**. So, the **figures in red translate, approximately, as follows**:

6.5 MMOL/L = 252 mg/dl (supposedly dangerous levels)

5.5 MMOL/L = 213 mg/dl (supposedly borderline)

4.5 MMOL/L = 174 mg/dl (supposedly "least likely" to incur heart attacks)

Death rates (the black numbers and line) are per 100,000 population.

Study those World Health Organization numbers, and draw your own conclusions.

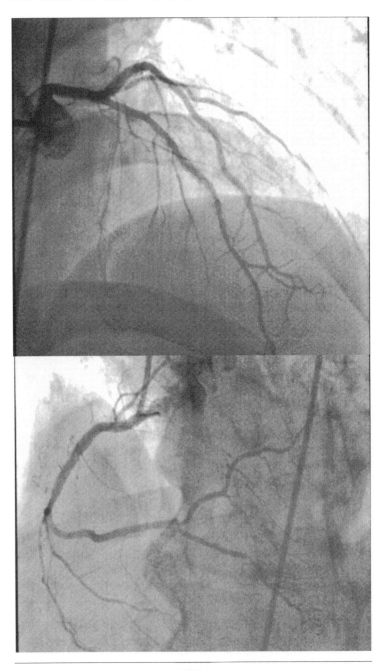

Printed in Great Britain
by Amazon.co.uk, Ltd.,
Marston Gate.